Intermittent Fasting 16:8 Cookbook

Delightful and Easy Recipes for a Rapid Weight Loss and Optimal Health

Melanie Roy

the reader will render any resulting actions solely under their purview. There are no scenarios in which the publisher or the original author of this work can be in any fashion deemed liable for any hardship or damages that may befall them after undertaking information described herein.

Additionally, the information in the following pages is intended only for informational purposes and should thus be thought of as universal. As befitting its nature, it is presented without assurance regarding its prolonged validity or interim quality. Trademarks that are mentioned are done without written consent and can in no way be considered an endorsement from the trademark holder.

TABLE OF CONTENTS

INTRODUCTION

What is intermittent fasting?

It is a diet that includes a fast of 16 hours or less. This means that every user plans a fasting period in their everyday life. This can vary in length depending on the type of intermittent fasting. Intermittent fasting takes into account that you are not allowed to consume solid foods for a certain period of time and then eat normally for a predetermined period of time. But what actually happens when you are interested in intermittent fasting yourself.

Types of intermittent Fasting

The classic and best-known form is **16:8** intermittent fasting. It includes a fasting period of 16 hours, which is best observed overnight. The 8 hours refer to the time in which food can be consumed.

All you have to do is figure out a period when you would like to consume your normal three meals. Say, for example, you have your dinner by 8 p.m. The next meal has to be consumed only after 12 noon the next day. You will have to skip breakfast and go for lunch instead. It is your choice to have 3 meals or limit it to two, i.e., lunch, snack and dinner or lunch and dinner in the next 8 hours.

This intermittent fast is easier to adopt for those who are accustomed to skipping breakfast. All you have to do is ensure you do not consume anything in the fasting hours. You are, however, allowed to have liquids. You can have any type of liquid including juices; fruit infused water, coconut water, etc. Just make sure you keep a tab on the calorie level and avoid sugary drinks or those with calories.

Fasting has been used for religious, cultural, and spiritual purposes throughout history and around the world. Fasting has become popular among those who want to lose weight without having to give up specific foods as a result of the media coverage provided to diets like the **5:2** diet in recent years. IF focuses on the periods of time that we don't feed – what we term "fasting." The frequency and length of these fasting periods are determined by the type of diet followed and the schedule of the person. The following are some examples of common IF eating patterns: Choosing a time frame for eating each day and abstaining from eating outside of it. The 5:2 diet includes consuming just 25% of a regular calorie intake (500 kcals for women, 600 kcals for men) on two days per week and eating regularly on the remaining five.

Fasting 20:4: With this method, the user needs a period of getting used to, because the fasting period is extremely long at 20 hours. In the remaining 4 hours you can easily eat whatever you want. The success relates to the fact that you ingest larger amounts during these 4 hours, which in turn are digested and used in the 20 hours.

Fasting 36:12: In this type of fasting, the method is based on fasting every other day. That is, you eat normally from 8 a.m. to 8 p.m. and fast the night and the entire day after that. This method is only for experienced users.

Fasting 14:8: This method is the counterpart to the 16/8 method and is actually reserved for women. With this method it has to be clearly stated that the fasting time is 14 hours and the meal time is 8 hours, which of course does not add up to 24 hours. Even so, this method is recommended for women.

Warrior diet

The warrior diet is a rather simple form of intermittent fast. It can be considered as a beginner's intermittent fast. All you have to do is go for small portions of vegetables and fruit in the mornings. You then have a regular meal at night. There is no restriction on what you can consume for dinner. The warrior diet is so called because athletes and sportsmen trying to get fit follow this plan.

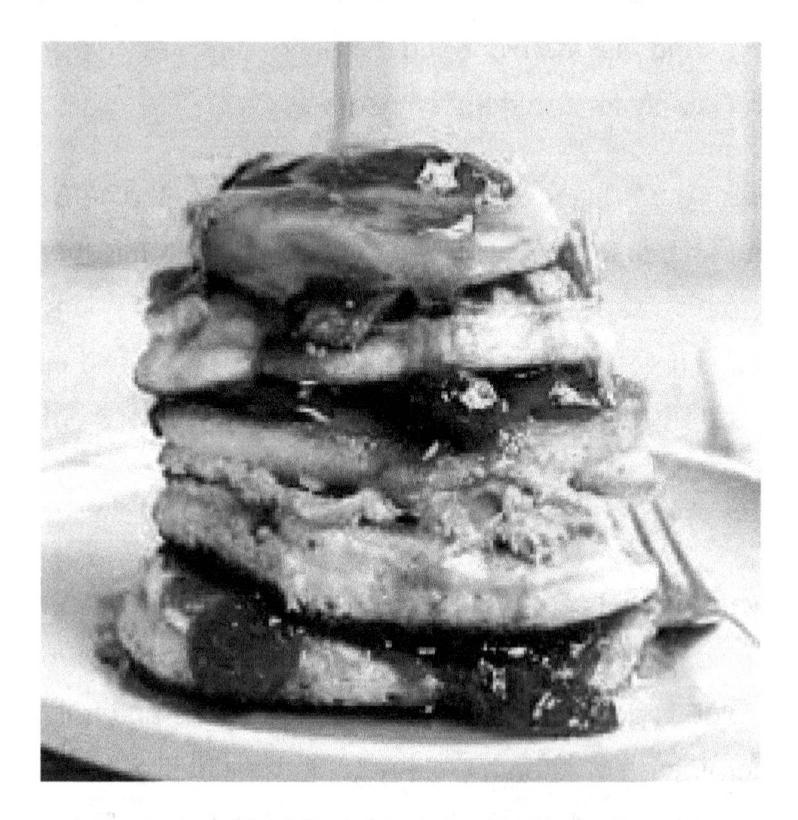

Breakfast Recipes

CHOCO CHIP WHEY WAFFLES

10 minutes

6 minutes

2 Servings

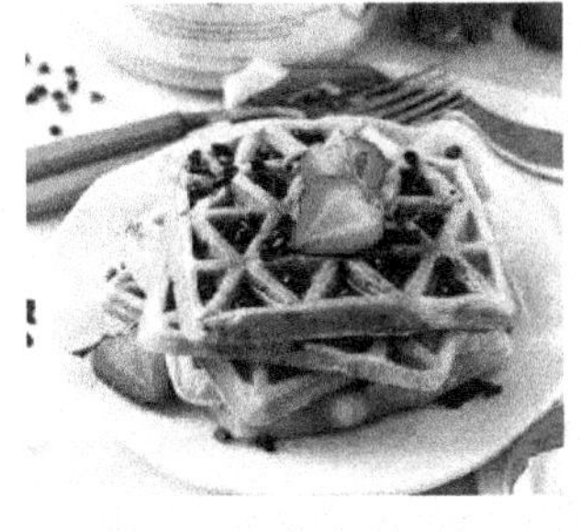

INGREDIENTS

- 2 tablespoons of organic coconut oil
- 2 tablespoons of coconut sugar
- 4 tablespoons of chocolate whey protein powder
- ⅓ cup of almond flour
- A pinch of salt
- ½ teaspoon of baking powder
- ½ cup of almond milk
- 2 eggs

COOKING STEPS

1. Mix all the ingredients in the blender to obtain a homogeneous paste.
2. Preheat your waffle iron. Pour the waffle batter into the iron and bake each waffle for 3 minutes.

AVOCADOS ON TOASTED SPREADS

10 minutes

5 minutes

2 Servings

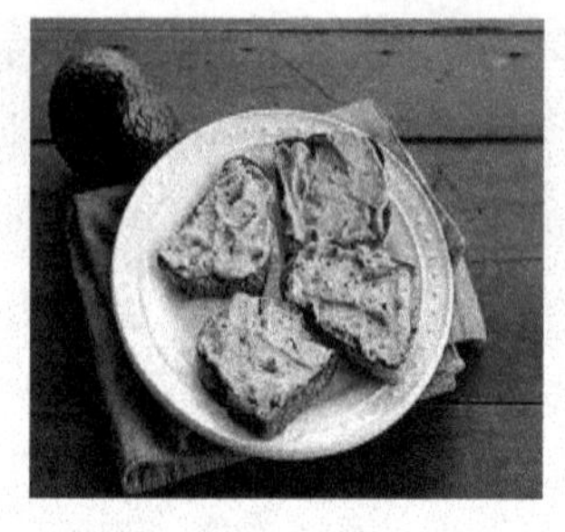

INGREDIENTS

- slice bread, gluten free
- ½ pc small avocado, thinly sliced
- 1 tablespoon of cream cheese
- 1 teaspoon of lemon juice
- Pinch of salt and pepper
- 1 teaspoon of chia seeds for garnish (optional)

COOKING STEPS

1. Lightly toast the slices of bread.
2. Carefully arrange the avocado slices on each slice of bread.
3. Drizzle with lemon juice. Spread the cream cheese.
4. Sprinkle with pepper and salt.
5. Garnish with garnish.

SCRAMBLED EGGS WITH SWISS CHARD

10 minutes

10 minutes

2 Servings

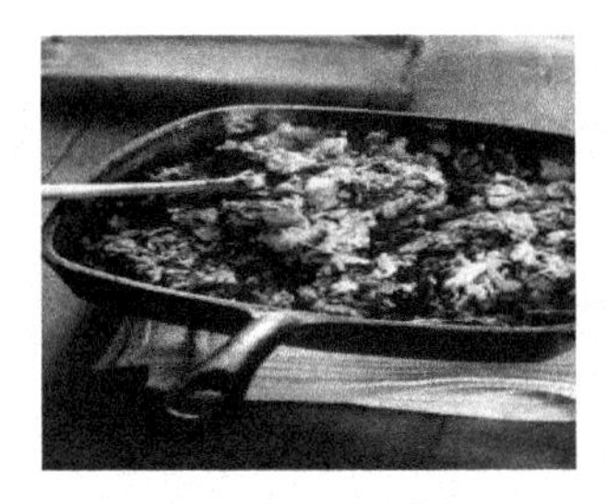

INGREDIENTS

- 1 teaspoon olive oil
- 2 eggs
- 4 tablespoons of milk
- 250g Swiss chard
- salt and pepper
- 1 red onion
- thyme
- 30g Gouda
- 1 red pepper

COOKING STEPS

1. Peel and wash the onion and cut into fine rings. Wash the peppers, cut in half lengthways, remove the seeds and chop finely.
2. Wash and chop the chard.
3. Put the eggs, salt, pepper, milk and chopped thyme in a bowl and mix together.
4. Heat the oil in a pan and sauté the onion, bell pepper and chard in it. Pour eggs over it.
5. Finely grate the Gouda cheese. Let the scrambled eggs set for 3 minutes.

ROLLS

20 minutes

40 minutes

10 Servings

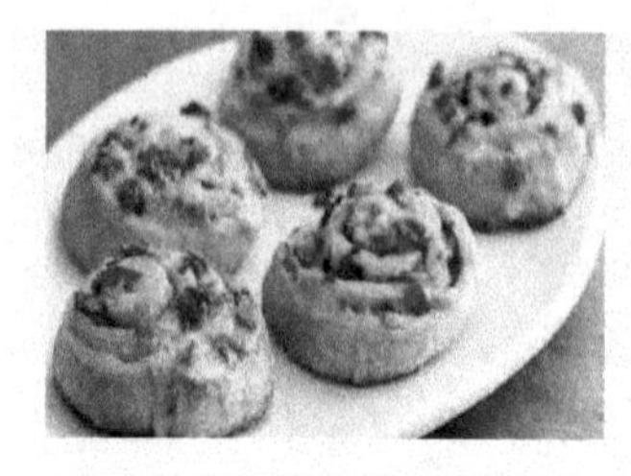

INGREDIENTS

- 170g flaxseed, ground
- 150g gluten
- 60g almond flour
- 50g pumpkin seeds
- 20g sunflower seeds, roughly chopped
- 10g dry yeast
- 2 teaspoons of salt
- 1 teaspoon bread spice
- 330ml lukewarm water
- Sesame seeds, for sprinkling

COOKING STEPS

1. Preheat oven to 180 degrees.
2. Mix the linseed, gluten, yeast, almond flour, salt and bread spices in a bowl.
3. Add lukewarm water and knead into a solid mass. Add the pumpkin and sunflower seeds and knead well again.
4. Line the baking sheet with parchment paper. Shape the dough into 10 rolls of the same size and place on the
5. tray. Sprinkle the rolls with sesame seeds and then cover and leave for 40 minutes.
6. Bake the rolls in the oven for 30 minutes.

FRUITY SEMOLINA PORRIDGE

10 minutes

15 minutes

2 Servings

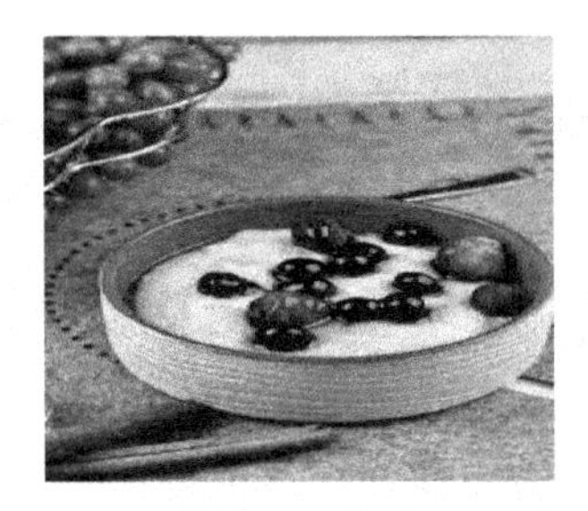

INGREDIENTS

- 3 tbsp semolina
- 200 ml plant milk (e.g. almond milk)
- 1 tbsp maple syrup
- 100 ml coconut cream
- ½ teaspoon cinnamon
- 125 g strawberries
- 1 tbsp cornstarch
- 125 g rhubarb

COOKING STEPS

1. Put the almond milk, coconut cream, semolina, maple syrup and cinnamon in a saucepan.
2. Mix the ingredients together and let the whole thing cook (and stir) until it has a good consistency.
3. Wash the strawberries and rhubarb and then cut them into small pieces.
4. The rhubarb and strawberries also need to be heated in a saucepan with a little water.
5. Mix the cornstarch with approx. 2 tablespoons of water and then also add to the saucepan.
6. As soon as the consistency becomes a little thicker, the compote is ready.

BANANA PANKAKES

15 minutes

10 minutes

4 Servings

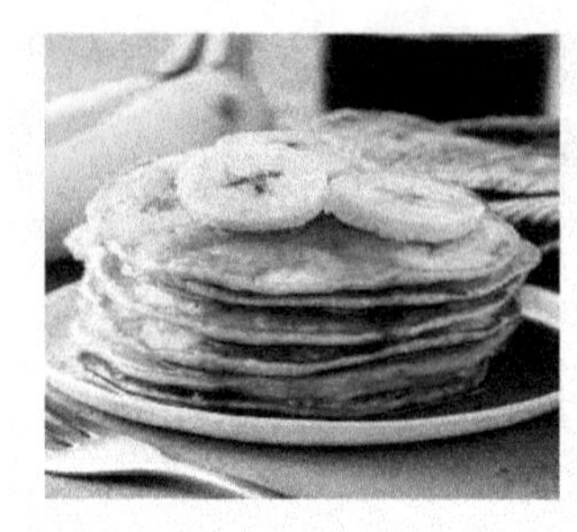

INGREDIENTS

- 1 ripe banana
- 150 g flour (wheat or spelled)
- 250 ml plant milk (e.g. almond milk)
- 1 teaspoon baking powder
- 1 pinch of salt
- 1 teaspoon cinnamon some oil

COOKING STEPS

1. Mix the flour, cinnamon, baking powder and salt carefully together in a bowl.
2. Mash the banana with a fork or spoon.
3. Mix the mashed banana with the vegetable milk and then add the dry ingredients.
4. Mix everything together well and then fry the pancakes in a pan with oil.
5. After about 4 minutes, turn the pancake over and fry for another 4 minutes.

CHEESE AND HAM OMELETTE

5 minutes

10 minutes

1 Servings

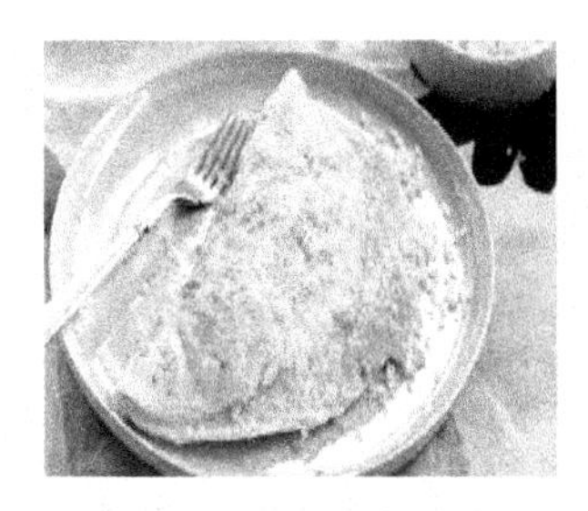

INGREDIENTS

- 1 tomato
- 2 eggs
- 2 tbsp grated cheese
- 1 teaspoon butter
- 1 tbsp milk
- 2 slices of cooked ham
- 1 tbsp parsley salt and pepper

COOKING STEPS

1. Wash the tomatoes and then cut them into small pieces and cut the ham into thin strips.
2. The eggs are then mixed with the milk and then seasoned with salt and pepper.
3. After that, the mixture is poured into a pan with butter.
4. Let the egg fry until it sets.
5. Turn the heat down a little and add the cheese, ham, tomatoes and parsley and let it sizzle for half a minute.
6. After half a minute, the omelette can be taken out and eaten.

VEGETARIAN VARIETY WITH PENUT PASTE

15 minutes

15 minutes

1 Servings

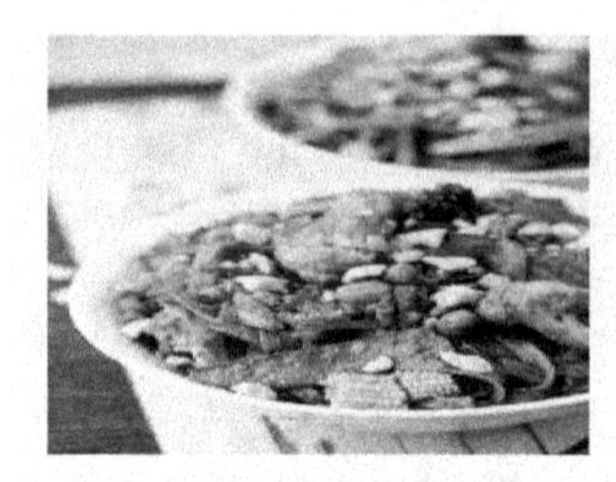

INGREDIENTS

- 1 small onion bulb, thinly sliced
- ¾ cup broccoli, cut into wedges
- 1 pc small carrot, cut into wedges
- ½ pc green pepper, thinly sliced
- 5 mushrooms, cut into wedges
- A pinch of salt, pepper and chili powder
- 2 tablespoons of peanut butter, dairy free
- 2 tbsp. soy sauce, gluten free

COOKING STEPS

1. Pour a little water into a heated pan and cook the onions until they are transparent.
2. Add the broccoli, carrot, pepper and mushrooms.
3. Cook 10 minutes until tender. (Add water if the pan is too dry).
4. Season the vegetables with a pinch of salt, pepper and chili.
5. For the sauce, mix the peanut butter with the soy sauce, agave syrup and 3 tablespoons of water.
6. To serve, stir in the red cabbage.
7. Garnish the dish with the sauce.

- 1 tablespoon of agave syrup (or honey), gluten free
- ¼ cup red cabbage, thinly sliced

FARMER'S BREAKFAST

10 minutes

20 minutes

2 Servings

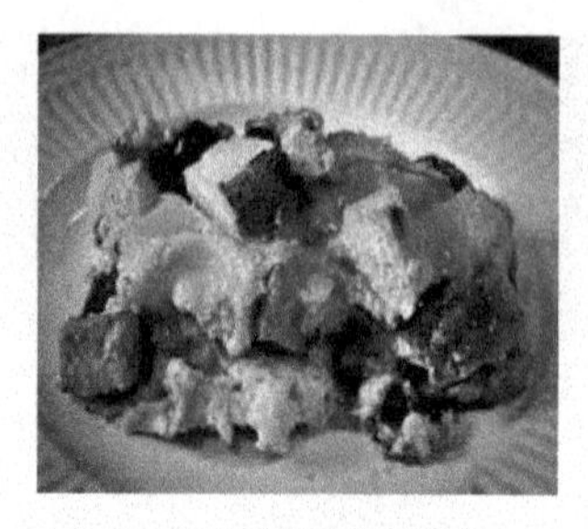

INGREDIENTS

- 2 tbsp olive oil
- 100g red peppers
- 100g eggplant
- 4 eggs
- 1 pinch of paprika powder
- 1 tbsp coriander, chopped
- 2 tbsp natural yogurt
- 4 flat breads
- salt and pepper

COOKING STEPS

1. Wash, peel and finely dice the eggplant. Wash the peppers, cut in half lengthways, remove the seeds and finely chop.
2. Heat the oil in a pan, add the peppers and eggplants and sauté. Season with salt and pepper. Simmer for 7 minutes.
3. Whisk eggs with paprika, salt and pepper. Pour over the pepper mixture and let it set until the egg mixture has set.
4. Wash and finely chop the coriander. Sprinkle over the farmer's breakfast and serve with yogurt and flatbreads.

QUARK BUNS

15 minutes

20 minutes

6 Servings

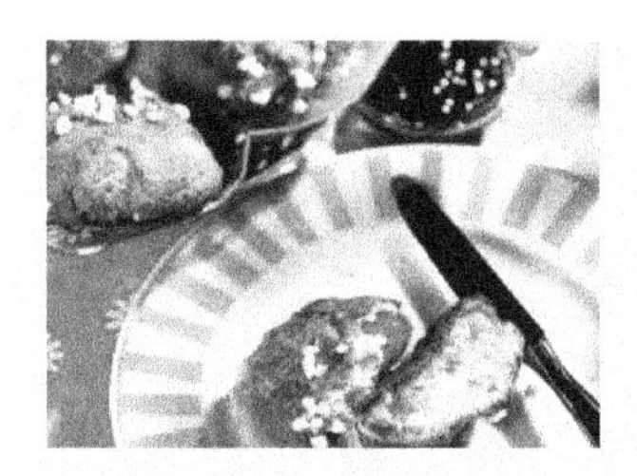

INGREDIENTS

- 200 g quark
- 4 eggs
- 125 g cream cheese
- 50 g chia seeds
- 300 g ground almonds
- 25 g of flaxseed
- 1 teaspoon baking powder
- salt and pepper of baking powder

COOKING STEPS

1. Puree the flax seeds with the chia seeds in a blender until a floury consistency is obtained.
2. Put all the remaining ingredients in a bowl and mix them together well. Finally, add the chia and flax seeds and season
3. the mixture with salt and pepper. Now the dough has to rest for about 15 minutes.
4. After the time, 6 rolls can be formed from the dough. It must be ensured that the rolls have enough space, otherwise they will stick together.
5. Depending on your needs, seeds can also be placed on the rolls.
6. Set the oven to top and bottom heat and 175 ° and leave the rolls in the oven for about 30 minutes.

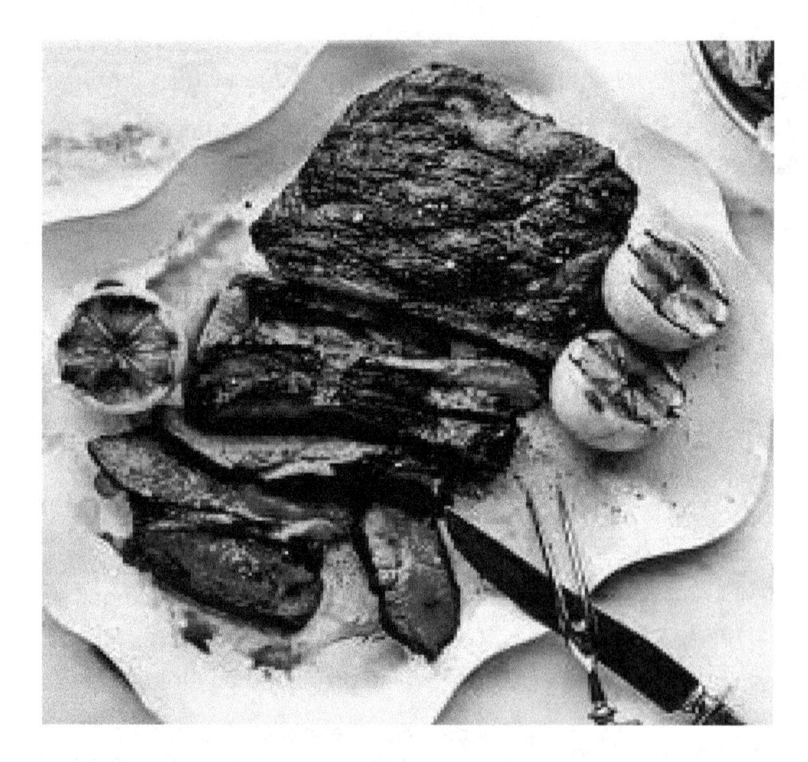

Meat Recipes

CHICKEN WITH BROCCOLI

10 minutes

20 minutes

2 Servings

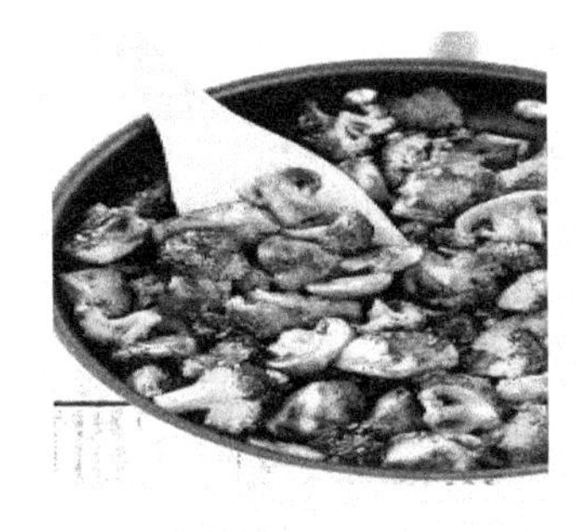

INGREDIENTS

- 200 g green asparagus
- 500 g broccoli
- 600 g chicken breast fillet
- 400 ml vegetable stock
- 1 clove of garlic
- ½ lemon
- 3 tbsp flour Chicken Seasoning
- salt and pepper

COOKING STEPS

1. Wash the meat and cut it into pieces.
2. Mix 2 tablespoons of flour with 1 tablespoon of chicken seasoning and turn the meat in it.
3. Wash off the broccoli and asparagus and cook as usual.
4. Put some oil in a pan and fry the meat in it until it turns brown.
5. The meat comes out of the pan and the vegetables come in.
6. Deglaze with the vegetable stock and squeeze in the clove of garlic.
7. Put a lid on and let it simmer for a few minutes.
8. Add the tablespoon of flour to the pan and let it simmer.
9. Finally, put the meat back in and let the lemon juice and the whole thing warm up. Just add salt and pepper to taste and it's ready.

BEEF PAN

10 minutes

40 minutes

2 Servings

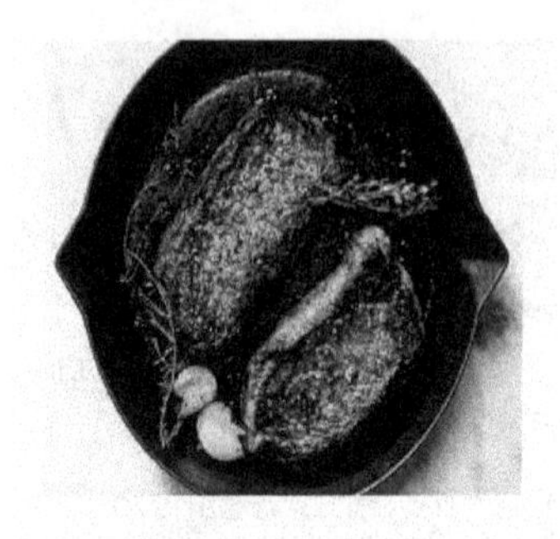

INGREDIENTS

- 200 g tomatoes
- 6 peppers
- 1 onion
- 1 clove of garlic
- 1 chili pepper
- 10 g parsley
- 600 g beef 750 ml of broth 20 g tomato paste
- 2 tbsp paprika powder Salt, pepper, coriander,
- caraway seeds

COOKING STEPS

1. Chop the bell pepper, onion and garlic into small pieces. Finely chop the chili and cut the tomatoes in half.
2. Wash the meat and cut into strips. Put the oil in a pan and fry the meat for a few minutes and then remove it from the pan.
3. Add the onion, chili and garlic. Then add the tomato paste and paprika powder and sauté for a minute.
4. Add the broth, peppers, tomatoes and meat to the pan and season with spices.
5. Let the whole thing simmer for 30 minutes. Finally, just add the parsley.

BEEF KALE PATTIES

10 minutes

40 minutes

2 Servings

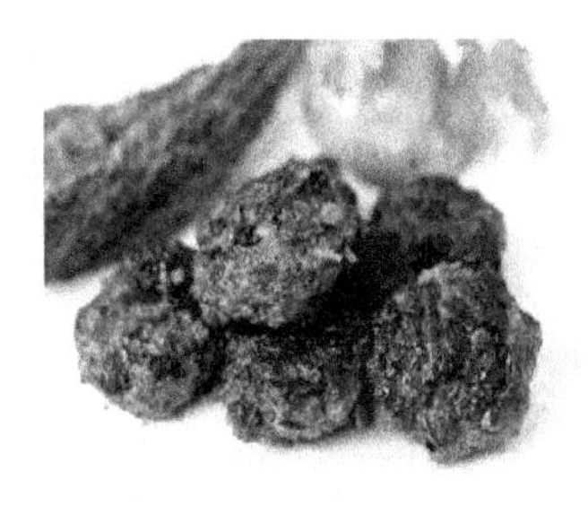

INGREDIENTS

- 1 lb Ground beef
- 1 cup Fresh kale, finely chopped
- 1 Egg, beaten
- 1 tbsp. Almond flour
- 1 tbsp Olive oil

Spices

- ½ tsp. Dried rosemary
- ½ tsp. Dried oregano
- 1 tsp Sea salt
- ½ tsp. Black pepper
- 1 cup Water

COOKING STEPS

1. Combine the flour, egg, kale, and beef in a bowl. Mix with your hand until mixed well. Add flour and all spices. Mix and shape about 8 patties, about 2-inch in diameter.
2. Grease a fitting springform pan with olive oil. Add the patties and set aside.
3. Pour 1-cup water in the inner pot of the IP. Position a trivet on the bottom and place the pan on top.
4. Cover and press Manual and cook on High-pressure for 15 minutes.
5. Do a quick release and open the pot.
6. Cool and serve.
7. Optionally, brown the patties on Sauté mode for 1 minute on both sides

BEEF CHUCK ROAST

10 minutes

35 minutes

3 Servings

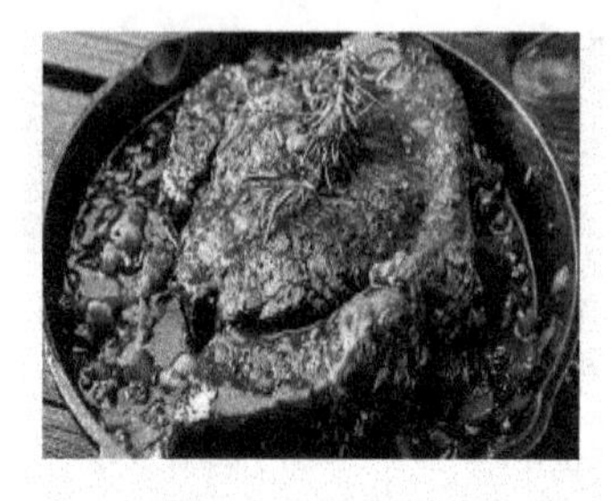

INGREDIENTS

- 1 ½ lb. Beef chuck roast - cut into bite-sized pieces
- 2 Garlic cloves, minced
- ½ tbsp Butter
- 1 cup Beef broth
- ½ cup Tomatoes,diced
- ½ Onion, chopped
- ½ tsp Black pepper.
- Sea salt to taste

COOKING STEPS

1. Melt the butter in the IP over Sauté setting.
2. Add onions and garlic and cook for 3 to 4 minutes or until onions are translucent.
3. Add meat and cook for 5 minutes on each side.
4. Add tomatoes and all the spices. Pour in the broth and cover with the lid.
5. Press manual and cook for 25 minutes on High.
6. Once cooked, release pressure naturally.
7. Open the pot and transfer the meat to a serving plate.
8. Enjoy.

PAPRIKA SAUCE WITH SHREDDED MEAT

10 minutes

30 minutes

2 Servings

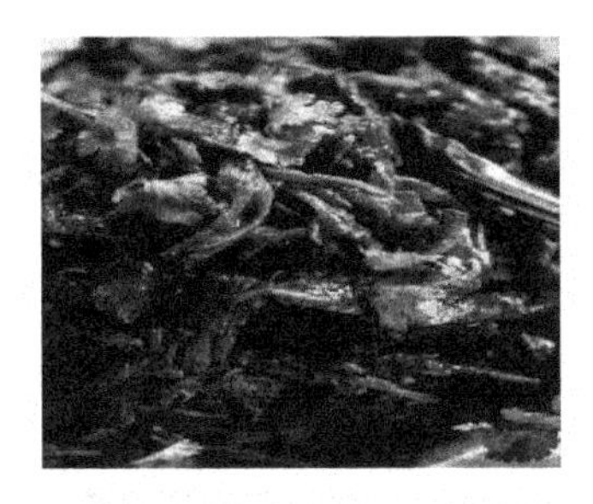

INGREDIENTS

- 125 ml of cream
- 2 tbsp tomato paste
- 125 ml of broth
- 2 onions
- 2 peppers
- 500 g pork schnitzel
- 2 tbsp flour
- 1 tbsp paprika powder
  salt and pepper

COOKING STEPS

1. Wash and chop the meat.
2. Mix the flour with salt and pepper and wilt the meat in it. Chop the onions and peppers too.
3. Heat the oil in a pan and add the meat. Add the onion and paprika and season with paprika powder.
4. Add the broth and cream and let it cook for about 20 minutes with the lid on.
5. Stir in the tomato paste and season with salt and pepper.

PORK FILLET WITH SAGE POTATOES

10 minutes

45 minutes

2 Servings

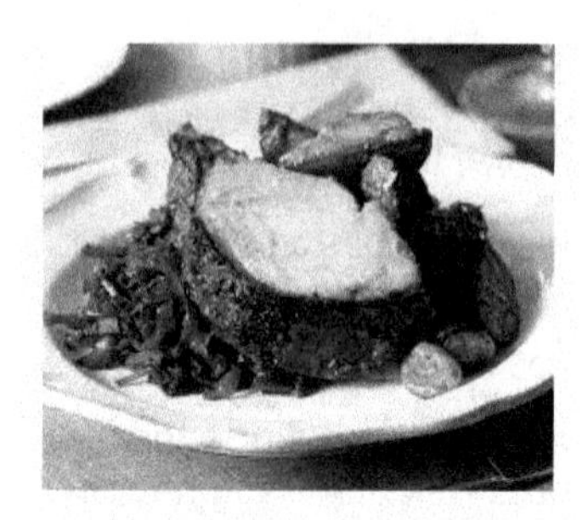

INGREDIENTS

- 280 g pork tenderloin
- 500 g potatoes
- 200 g rhubarb
- 50 g celery 5 g of sage 5 g parsley
- 150 g crème fraîche
- 100 ml of water salt and pepper

COOKING STEPS

1. Preheat the oven to 200 ° C top and bottom heat. Finely chop the parsley and sage.
2. Wash and quarter the potatoes. Then place them in a bowl with the sage and add 1 tablespoon of oil. Then place the potatoes on a baking sheet and bake in the oven for 25-30 minutes.
3. Cut off the ends of the celery and rhubarb, and peel the rhubarb as well. Then cut the two ingredients into small pieces. Heat the oil in a pan and add the celery and rhubarb and fry for 3 minutes.
4. Wash the meat and then divide it into 4 equal pieces. Put the meat in a pan and fry for 5 minutes on each side.
5. Add 100 ml of water with a little sugar to the rhubarb and let it simmer for about 5 minutes. Turn the heat down and add the crème fraîche, salt and pepper.
6. Finally, put the potatoes, sauce and meat on plates and enjoy.

GARLICKY PORK SHOULDER

10 minutes

4 hours

8 Servings

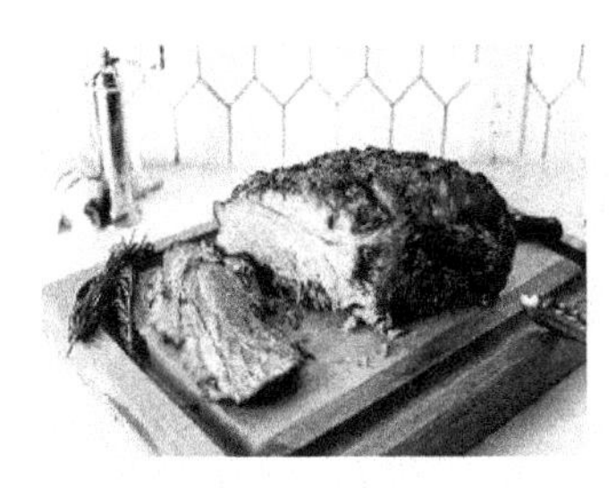

INGREDIENTS

- head garlic, peeled and crushed
- ¼ C. fresh rosemary, minced 2 tbsp. fresh lemon juice
- tbsp. balsamic vinegar
- 1 (4-lb.) pork shoulder

COOKING STEPS

1. In a bowl, add all the ingredients except pork shoulder and mix well.
2. In a large roasting pan, place the pork shoulder and generously coat with the marinade.
3. With a large plastic wrap, cover the roasting pan and refrigerate to marinate for at least 1-2 hours.
4. Remove the roasting pan from refrigerator.
5. Remove the plastic wrap from roasting pan and keep in room temperature for 1 hour.
6. Preheat the oven to 2750 F.
7. Place the roasting pan into oven and roast for about 6 hours.
8. Remove from the oven and place pork shoulder onto a cutting board for about 30 minutes.
9. With a sharp knife, cut the pork shoulder into desired size slices and serve.

SIMPLE EVER RIB ROAST

15 minutes

1 hour

12 Servings

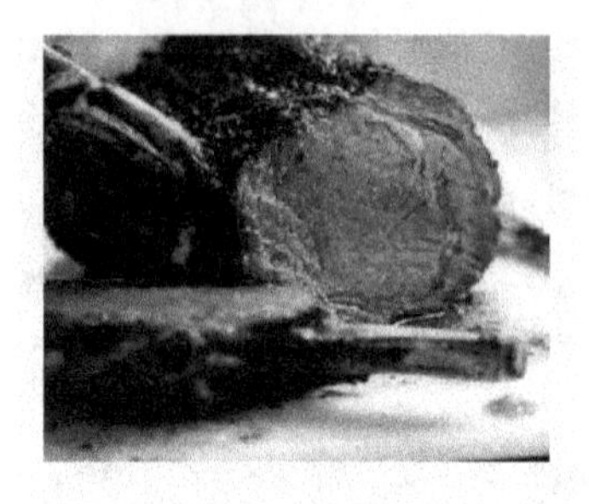

INGREDIENTS

- 10 garlic cloves, minced
- 2 tsp. dried thyme, crushed 2 tbsp. olive oil
- Salt and freshly ground black pepper, to taste
- 1 (10-lb.) grass-fed prime rib roast

COOKING STEPS

1. In a bowl, mix together all the ingredients except rib roast.
2. In a large roasting pan, place the rib roast, fatty side up. Coat the rib roast with garlic mixture evenly.
3. Set aside to marinate at the room temperature for at least 1 hour.
4. Preheat the oven to 5000 F. Roast for about 20 minutes.
5. Now, reduce the temperature of oven to 3250 F.
6. Roast for 65-75 minutes.
7. Remove from oven and place the roast onto a cutting board for about 10-15 minutes before slicing.
8. With a sharp knife cut the rib roast in desired sized slices and serve.

MARINATED CHICKEN WITH DIP

10 minutes

30 minutes

4 Servings

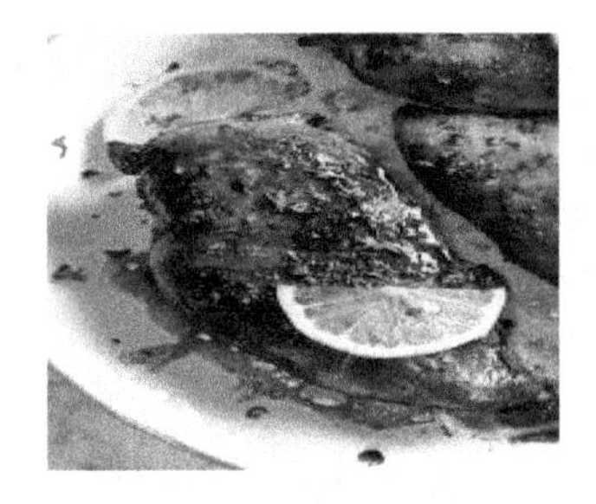

INGREDIENTS

- 300 g frozen peas
- 2 cloves of garlic
- 3 stalks of mint
- 4 chicken fillets
- 3 tbsp yogurt
- 3 tbsp mustard
- 2 tbsp soy sauce
- 2 tbsp honey
- 3 tbsp lemon juice
- 4 tbsp olive oil
- Salt, pepper, sugar

COOKING STEPS

1. Mix the mustard, soy sauce, honey, 1 tablespoon lemon juice and 2 tablespoons olive oil in a bowl.
2. Wash the meat and add it as well. Season with salt and pepper and put in the fridge for 30 minutes.
3. Put the peas in boiling water and cook for 3 minutes.
4. Pluck the leaves from the mint, chop the garlic and then puree the peas, mint and garlic together with the lemon juice.
5. Then mix in the yogurt and 2 tablespoons of olive oil and season the whole thing.
6. Put the meat in a pan and fry for 10 minutes.
7. Finally, just place the dip and the meat on plates and serve.

DUCK BREAST WITH PROSCIUTTO

10 minutes

50 minutes

4 Servings

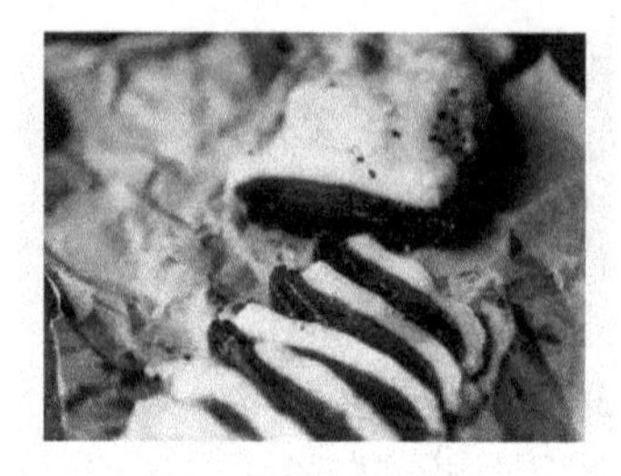

INGREDIENTS

- 1 lb Duck breasts
- 1 Shallot, finely chopped
- 2 Garlic cloves, crushed
- ½ cup Duck fat
- 4 cups Chicken broth
- 7 oz Prosciutto chopped
- 2 tbsp. Fresh parsley,chopped
- 3 tbsp. Apple
- 1 cup Cremini mushrooms
- 1 tbsp Orange zest

COOKING STEPS

1. Press Sauté and add the duck fat. Stir constantly and slowly melt the fat.
2. Add the garlic and shallots. Add the mushrooms and continue to cook until the liquid has evaporated.
3. Add the prosciutto and stir well. Briefly brown on all sides and press Cancel.
4. Add the meat into the pot and pour in the broth. Sprinkle with orange zest and spices.
5. Press Manual and cook 20 minutes on High pressure.
6. Once cooked release pressure naturally and open the lid.
7. Sprinkle with parsley and cover for 10 minutes before serving.

- 1 tsp. Sea salt
- ½ tsp. f White pepper reshly ground

BEEF STROGANOFF

10 minutes

20 minutes

4 Servings

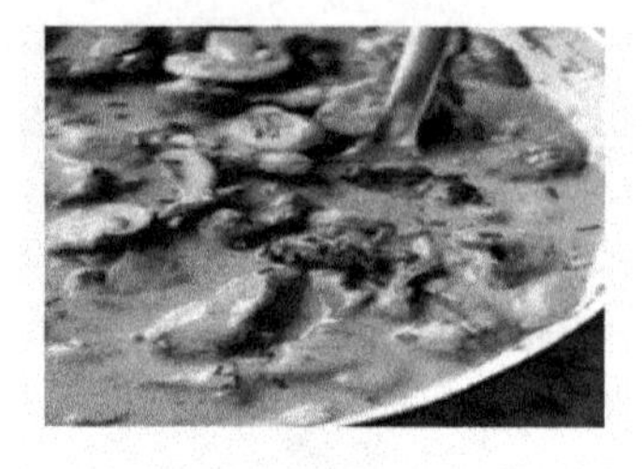

INGREDIENTS

- 1 Small onion, diced
- 2 Garlic cloves, crushed
- 2 Bacon rashers, diced
- 1 lb Beef Sirloin Steak (cut into ½ inch strips)
- 1 tsp. Smoked paprika
- 3 tbsp Tomato paste
- 1 cup Beef broth
- ½ lbs.Mushrooms . quartered
- ½ cup Sour cream

COOKING STEPS

1. Place all ingredients in the instant pot except the sour cream and stir to combine.
2. Place and lock the lid and manually set the cooking time to 20 minutes on high pressure.
3. Naturally release the pressure, and then stir in the sour cream.
4. Serve warm.

TUNA MEATBALLS

10 minutes

15 minutes

1 Servings

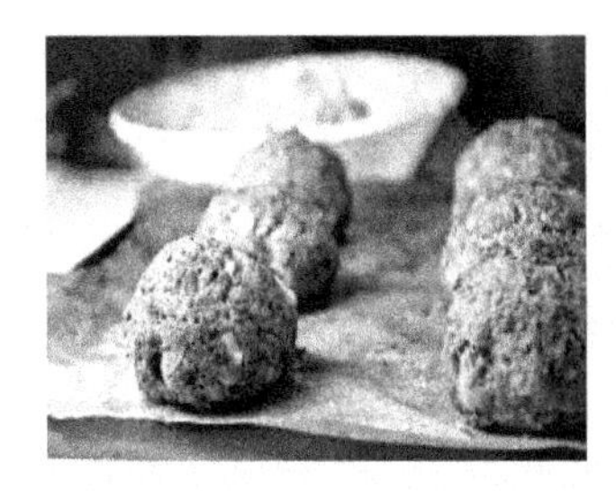

INGREDIENTS

- 1 spring onion
- 150 g beans (green)
- 1 shallot
- ½ bunch of parsley
- 120 g tuna
- 1 egg
- 2 teaspoons ajvar
- 3 tbsp oatmeal
- 1 tbsp apple cider vinegar
- 1 tbsp capers
- 1 teaspoon agave syrup salt and pepper

COOKING STEPS

1. Clean the beans, divide them in the middle, put them in boiling salted water and simmer for about 8 minutes.
2. Chop the shallot and add to the beans. Wash and chop the spring onions.
3. Pour off the juice from the tuna and then mix it with the spring onions, egg, ajvar, oat flakes, capers and salt and pepper.
4. Form meatballs out of this and put them in a pan with oil. Let fry for about 4 minutes.
5. Wash and chop the parsley. Mix with oil, vinegar and agave syrup and add to the beans.
6. Place the meatballs and the lettuce side by side and sprinkle with the parsley.

CHICKEN WITH BULGUR

10 minutes

40 minutes

2 Servings

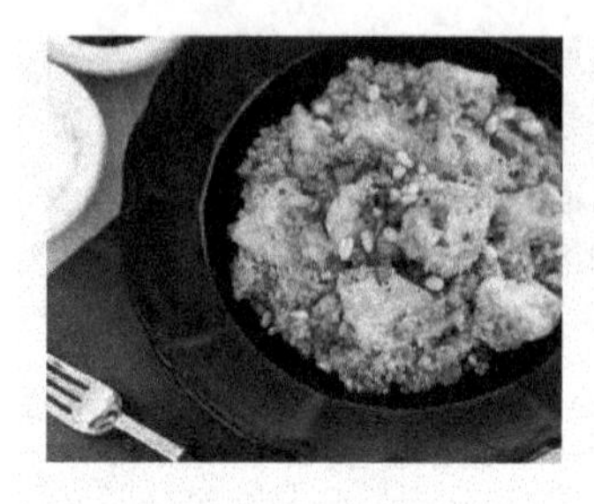

INGREDIENTS

- 100 g frozen beans (green)
- 1 onion
- 130 g mushrooms (brown)
- 1 stick of celery
- 2 carrots
- 1 clove of garlic
- 40 g bulgur
- 250 g chicken breast fillet
- 300 ml of chicken broth Salt, pepper, parsley

COOKING STEPS

1. Wash the meat, cut it into small pieces and season with salt and pepper. Put the bulgur in a colander and rinse it with water. Wash and chop the vegetables.
2. Heat the oil in a saucepan and add the meat. Add the vegetables and bulgur.
3. Pour in the broth and simmer for about 25 minutes.
4. Add the beans just before the end of the cooking time. Just season the whole thing with salt and pepper and add the parsley.

SUCCULENT PORK TENDERLOIN

20 minutes

1hour

4 Servings

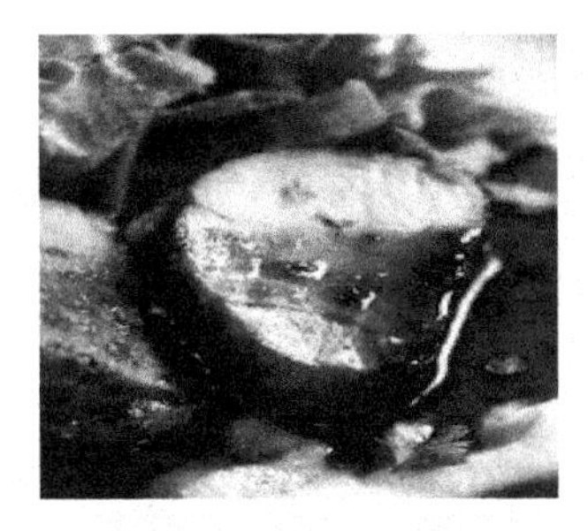

INGREDIENTS

- 1 lb. pork tenderloin
- 1 tbsp. unsalted butter
- 2 tsp. garlic, minced
- 2 oz. fresh spinach
- 4 oz. cream cheese, softened
- 1 tsp. liquid smoke
- Salt and black pepper

COOKING STEPS

1. Preheat the oven to 3500 F. Line casserole dish with a piece of the foil.
2. Arrange the pork tenderloin between 2 plastic wraps and with a meat tenderizer, pound until flat.
3. Carefully, cut the edges of tenderloin to shape into a rectangle.
4. In a large skillet, melt the butter over medium heat and sauté the garlic for about 1 minute.
5. Add the spinach, cream cheese, liquid smoke, salt and black pepper and cook for about 3-4 minutes.
6. Place the spinach mixture onto pork tenderloin about ½-inch from the edges.
7. Carefully roll tenderloin into a log and secure with toothpicks.
8. Arrange the tenderloin into the prepared casserole dish, seam-side down. Bake for about 1¼ hours.
9. Cut the tenderloin into desired sized slices and serve.

SALSA VERDE TURKEY BREAST

10 minutes

50 minutes

4 Servings

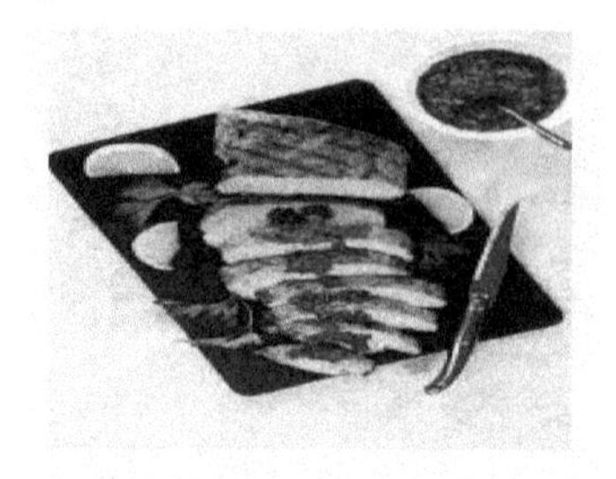

INGREDIENTS

- 2 Medium sized turkey breast, cut in half
- 1 Onion, sliced
- 3 cups Chicken broth

For the salsa Verde

- 1 cup Tomatillos, chopped
- ¼Fresh parsley chopped
- 1 Green chili, finely chopped
- 1 tsp Onion powder
- 2 Garlic cloves, crushed
- 3 tbsp Olive oil

COOKING STEPS

1. Combine the garlic powder, chili powder, onion powder, salt and cumin in a bowl. Mix well and set aside.
2. Rinse the meat under cold water and rub well with the spices.
3. Place at the bottom of the IP and pour in the chicken broth. Add the onions and seal the lid.
4. Press Poultry and cook on High for 15 minutes.
5. When cooked, release pressure naturally and open the lid. Remove the meat from the pot and set aside.
6. Remove the broth and press Sauté.
7. Grease the inner pot with olive oil and heat up.
8. Add garlic and green chili.
9. Cook for 2 to 3 minutes and then add the tomatillos along with remaining ingredients for the salsa.
10. Pour in about 3 tbsp. of the broth and simmer for 10 to 12 minutes. Stirring occasionally.
11. Press Cancel and remove the mixture from the pot. Transfer to a food processor and process until smooth.

- 1 tsp Salt
- ¼ tsp. Chili powder

For the rub

- 1 tsp Chili powder
- 2 tsp Garlic powder
- 1 tsp Onion powder
- 1 tsp Salt
- ½ tsp. Cumin powder

12. Drizzle over the meat and serve.

CAJUN BEEF

10 minutes

20 minutes

4 Servings

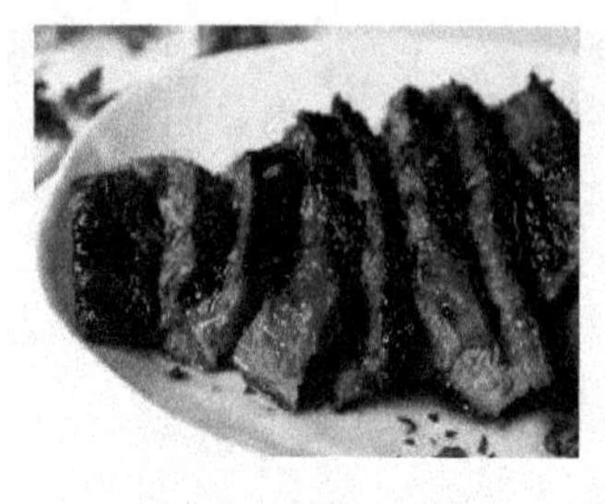

INGREDIENTS

- 1 tbsp. Cajun seasoning
- 12 ounces Mexican cheese blend
- 1 cup Beef broth
- 1 Ground beef pound
- 2 tbsp. Tomato paste
- 1 tbsp. Olive oil

COOKING STEPS

1. Press Sauté and heat the oil.
2. Add beef and cook until browned.
3. Stir in the tomato paste and seasoning.
4. Pour the broth over and close the lid.
5. Cook on High for 7 minutes.
6. Stir in the cheese and cook on High for 5 more minutes.
7. Do a quick pressure release.
8. Serve.

KALE PESTO WITH GNOCCHI

10 minutes

10 minutes

2 Servings

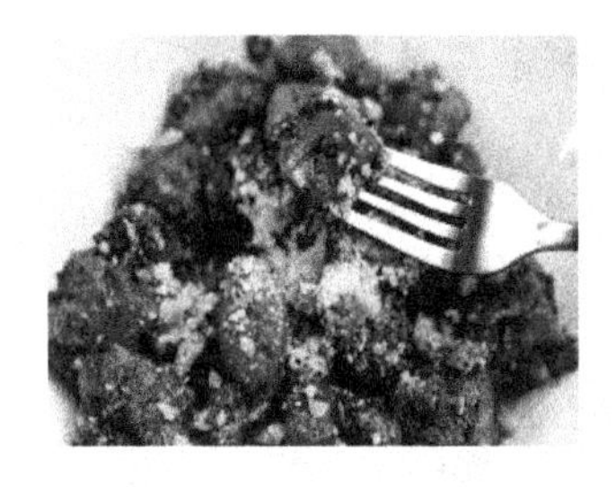

INGREDIENTS

- 400 g gnocchi
- 150 g kale
- 80 g ground almonds
- 2 cloves of garlic
- 4 teaspoons of lemon juice
- 6 slices of bacon
- 50 g parmesan cheese
- 60 ml of olive oil
- Salt, pepper, sugar

COOKING STEPS

1. Pluck the kale leaves and then wash the leaves. Dry the leaves again.
2. Chop the garlic and grate the parmesan. Put the kale, almonds and garlic in a blender and puree.
3. Always add a little oil and mix again. Finally add the parmesan and let the spices and pesto stand for now.
4. Preheat the oven to 220 ° C fan-assisted air.
5. Place the bacon on a baking sheet and put it in the oven for 8-12 minutes.
6. Take the whole thing out again and crumble into small pieces.
7. Prepare the gnocchi according to the instructions on the packet.
8. Then just put all the ingredients on a plate and refine with a little lemon juice.

CHICKEN WITH ZUCCHINI NOODLES

10 minutes

10 minutes

2 Servings

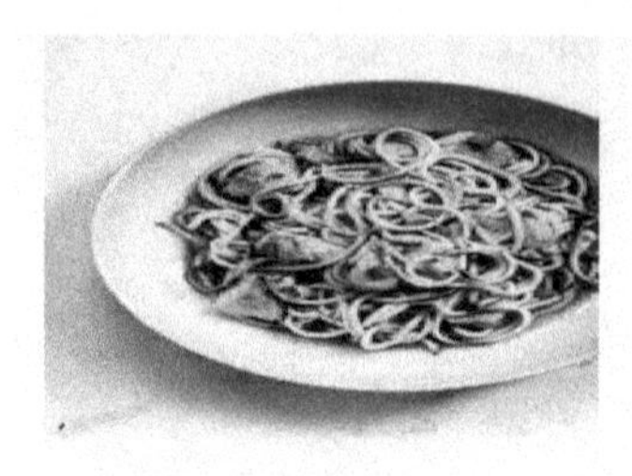

INGREDIENTS

- 100 g cherry tomatoes
- 1 zucchini
- 100 g of pasta
- 200 g of chicken
- 100 ml of cremefine
- 2 tbsp herb cream cheese some broth
- Salt, pepper, parsley, paprika

COOKING STEPS

1. Wash and chop the meat. Then the chicken must be seasoned as you like (paprika, salt, pepper, chili, etc.).
2. Meanwhile, put the pasta in boiling water and prepare according to the instructions on the packet.
3. Heat the oil in a pan and fry the chicken in it until it is cooked through. Remove the chicken.
4. Wash the zucchini and use a spiral peeler to make zucchini noodles.
5. The zucchini goes into the pan and needs to be sautéed. Then the tomatoes are added.
6. Add the cream cheese and then also the Cremefine and the broth. Bring the whole thing to the boil and then season.
7. Put the pasta and meat in the pan and mix everything together.

TURKEY BREAST IN CREAM CHEESE SAUCE

5 minutes

25 minutes

4 Servings

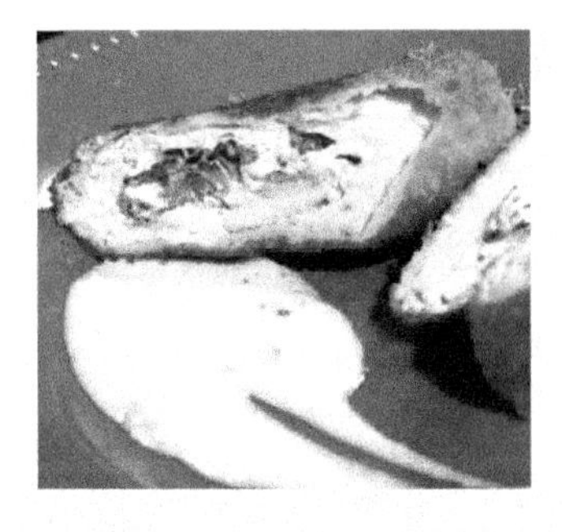

INGREDIENTS

- 500 potatos noodles
- 600 g turkey breast
- 300 g frozen peasg potato noodles
- 3 tablespoons cream cheese
- 4 stalks of mint
- 500 ml water
- 2 teaspoons vegetables stock
- Salt and pepper

COOKING STEPS

1. Wash, dry and cut the meat. Heat the oil in a pan and add the meat and fry for about 5 minutes.
2. Season with salt and pepper and take it out.
3. Now put the potato noodles in the pan and fry them for 5 minutes before they are also removed.
4. Add 500 ml of vegetable stock and the cream cheese and bring to the boil. Finally add the peas.
5. Wash off the mint and remove the leaves to chop them up.
6. Finally, add the meat, the potato noodles and the mint and mix everything together.

CHICKEN CHILI

15 minutes

35 minutes

8 Servings

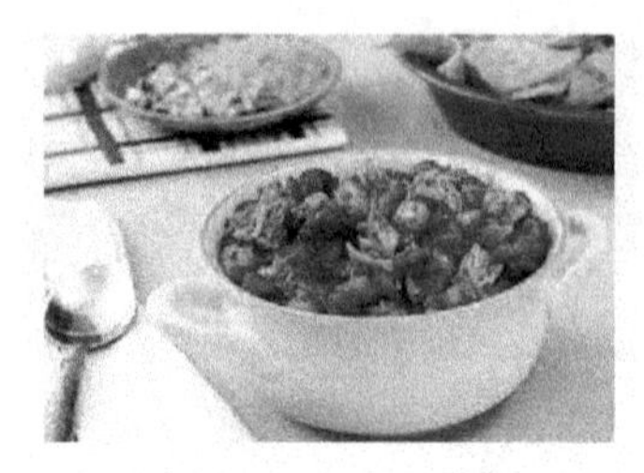

INGREDIENTS

- 8 (6 inches) corn tortillas
- 2 teaspoons vegetable oil
- 1 lb boneless chicken breast, diced
- 1 teaspoon ground cumin
- 1 cup poblano pepper, chopped
- 1/2 cup onion, chopped
- garlic clove, minced
- 2 (14 ounces) cans of reduced-fat chicken broth

COOKING STEPS

1. At 400 degrees F, preheat your oven.
2. Cut 4 the tortilla into ½ inch strips and toss them with 1 teaspoon oil.
3. Spread the tortillas on a baking sheet and bake for 12 minutes.
4. Grate the remaining tortillas into pieces and keep them aside.
5. Sauté chicken pieces with 1 teaspoon oil and cumin in a skillet for 5 minutes.
6. Transfer this prepared chicken to a plate and keep it aside.
7. Sauté garlic, onion and poblano peppers in the same skillet for 3 minutes.
8. Add grated tortillas, salsa, beans, broth and chicken, then cook for 15 minutes on a simmer.
9. Garnish with cilantro and baked tortillas. Serve warm.

- 2 (15 ounces) cans of pinto beans
- 1 cups salsa Verde
- 2 tablespoons cilantro, minced

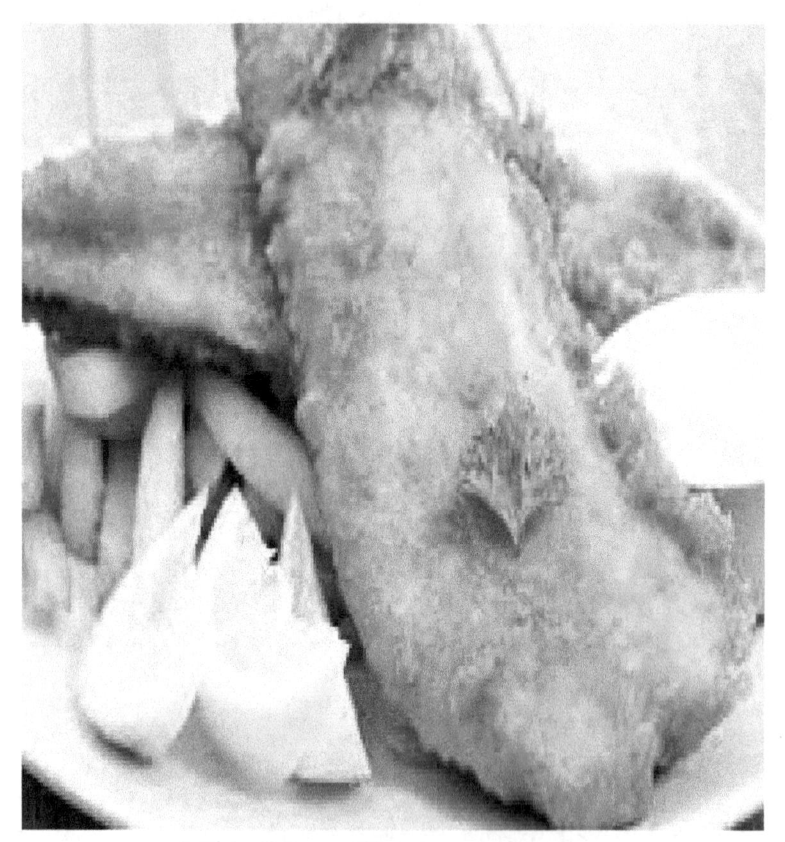

Fish Recipes

STEAMED SALMON AND SALAD BENTO BOX

10 minutes

0 minutes

2 Servings

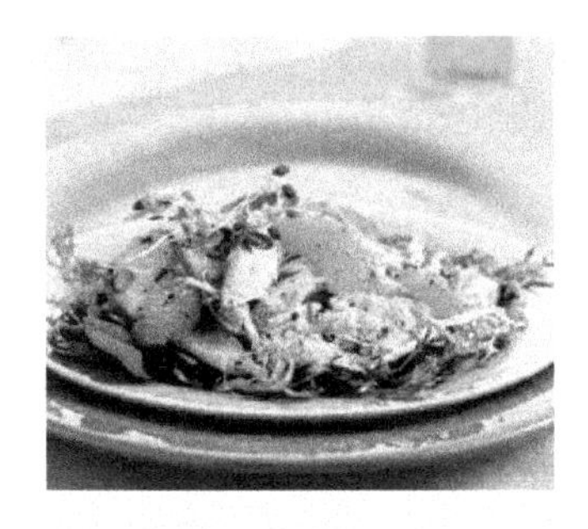

INGREDIENTS

- 2 heads of salad
- 1 cup of grated carrot
- ¼ cup cucumber, sliced
- 1 piece of green pepper, thinly sliced
- 4 cups marinara pasta, rinsed, drained and cooked for 2 minutes in boiling water
- ½ lb steamed salmon
- 2 lemons
- 2 eggs, boiled and sliced

COOKING STEPS

1. Divide the first eight ingredients evenly among two bento boxes.
2. Sprinkle the arrangements with chia seeds.
3. Mix the rest of the ingredients to make the sauce.
4. Pack the sauce separately.

- 1 teaspoon of chia seeds
- 4 tablespoons of yogurt, sugar free
- 1 teaspoon of turmeric powder
- ½ pc lemon, zest
- 2 tablespoons mint, minced
- Pinch of pepper

PERKY FISH FILLET & CHEESE COMBO

10 minutes

15 minutes

2 Servings

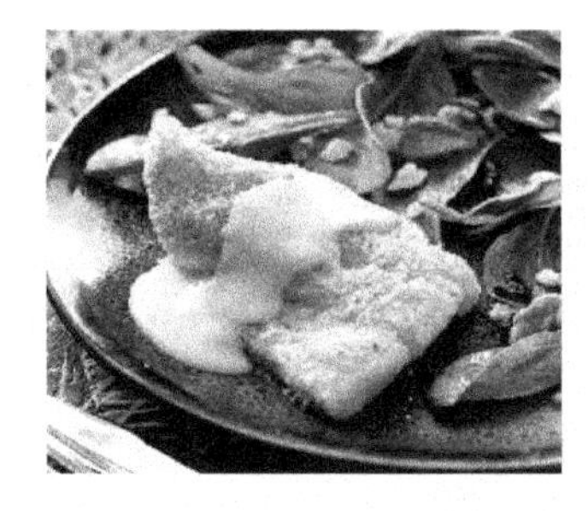

INGREDIENTS

- 1 tablespoon of olive oil
- 1 large potato, cooked and thinly sliced
- ¼ cup lean cottage cheese
- ½ teaspoon of herbs of your choice
- 3.5 oz. steamed herring fillet, halved
- ½ teaspoon of linseed oil or coconut oil
- Pinch of salt and pepper

COOKING STEPS

1. Heat a non-stick pan with olive oil.
2. Add the potato slices and cook for several minutes until golden brown.
3. Season the cottage cheese with salt, pepper and herbs of your choice.
4. Arrange the potatoes evenly between two plates.
5. Top with cheese and herring fillets. Garnish with a drizzle of linseed oil.

SALMON WITH SAUCE

5 minutes

15 minutes

2 Servings

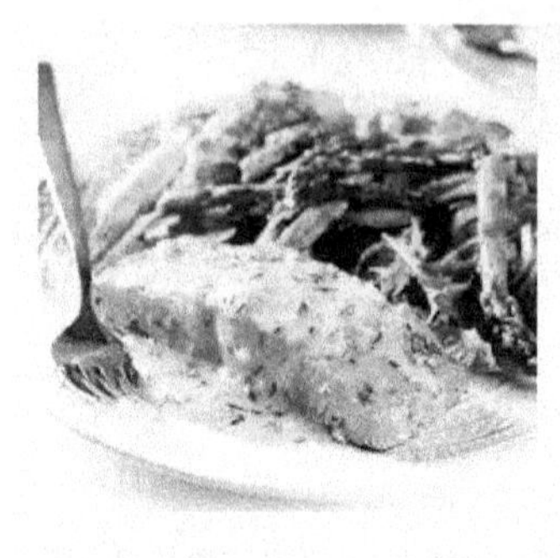

INGREDIENTS

- 1 1/2 lb. Salmon fillet
- 1 tbsp.Duck fat
- ¾ to 1 tsp Dried dill weed
- ¾ to 1 tsp Dried tarragon
- Salt and pepper to taste

Cream Sauce:

- 1/4 cup Heavy cream
- 2 tbsp. Butter -
- 1/2 tsp Dried dill weed
- 1/2 tsp Dried tarragon

COOKING STEPS

1. Slice the salmon in half and make 2 fillets. Season skin side with salt and pepper and meat of the fish with spices.
2. In a skillet, heat 1 tbsp. duck fat over medium heat.
3. Add salmon to the hot pan, skin side down.
4. Cook the salmon for about 5 minutes. When the skin is crisp, lower the heat and flip salmon.
5. Cook salmon on low heat for 7 to 15 minutes or until your desired doneness is reached.
6. Remove salmon from the pan and set aside.
7. Add spices and butter to the pan and let brown. Once browned, add cream and mix.
8. Top salmon with sauce and serve.

MAY PLAICE WITH LETTUCE

10 minutes

30 minutes

2 Servings

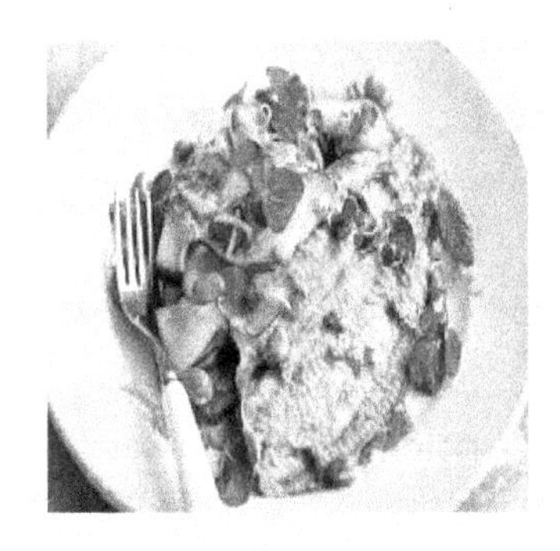

INGREDIENTS

- ½ lettuce
- 6 stems of chervil
- 3 tbsp white balsamic vinegar a bit of salt
- some pepper
- 2 teaspoons of liquid honey
- 3 tbsp oil
- 2 mash fillets
- 1 tbsp wheat flour
- ½ organic lemon 10 g butter

COOKING STEPS

1. Clean the lettuce and let it dry. Then wash the chervil and pluck the leaves. Chop these very finely.
2. For the salad dressing, please mix the balsamic vinegar with a little water and mix the spices and honey.
3. Add the chervil and stir everything together. Stir in a little oil.
4. Rinse the fish and season well. Then turn in the flour and knock off excess flour.
5. Heat the oil in a pan and fry the fish halves in it.
6. Wash the lemon with hot water and then cut it into slices.
7. Chop the lettuce leaves a little and mix with the salad sauce. Then arrange the plate with the salad and the fish.
8. Put the butter in a pan, heat it and pour it over the fish. Garnish with lemon and arrange everything.

SALMON GRILLED WITH FENNEL

10 minutes

20 minutes

2 Servings

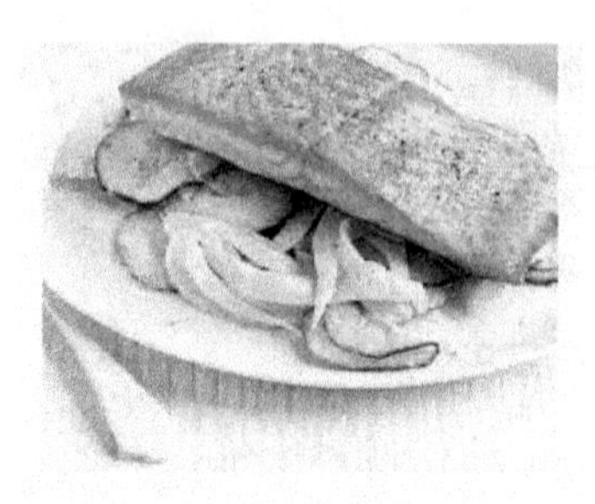

INGREDIENTS

- 500 g fennel bulb
- 100 ml classic vegetable stock
- 200 salmon fillet
- 2 tablespoons of oil
- 15 g red currants
- 125 g onions
- A bit of salad
- Some pepper

COOKING STEPS

1. Firstly, wash the fennel bulbs and separate the green. But don't throw it away.
2. Then wash the tubers and cut them into slices.
3. Put the vegetable stock in a saucepan and cook the fennel in this saucepan for 8 minutes.
4. Prepare the salmon and use a pan with oil or a grill pan. Fry the salmon on all sides for 3 minutes.
5. Clean the berries and set aside 1 tablespoon of the berries.
6. Wash the spring onions and cut into rings. Add the currants and spring onions to the fennel and cook for 2 minutes.
7. Then salt and pepper the vegetables.
8. Hen chop the fennel greens and serve with the salmon and vegetables.

FISH AND VEGETABLE PAN

10 minutes

15 minutes

2 Servings

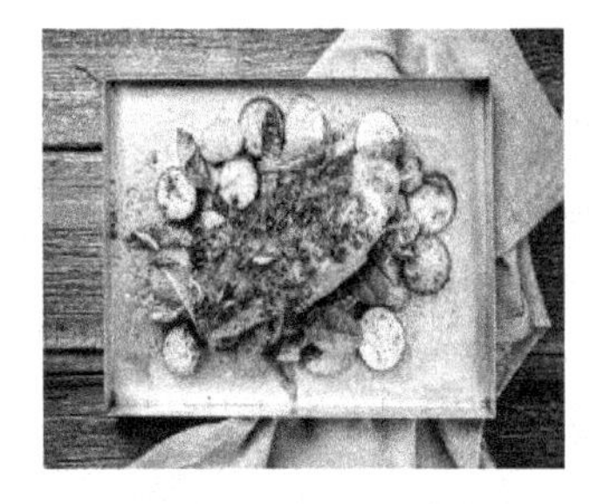

INGREDIENTS

- 300 g fish fillet
- 4 spring onions 100 g sugar peas
- 2 zucchini
- 200 g mushrooms
- 2 teaspoons of olive oil
- 300 g tomatoes with basil
- 1 bunch of chives
- 4 pinches of salt
- 4 pinches of pepper

COOKING STEPS

1. Please rinse the fish fillet and cut it into large cubes.
2. Then clean the spring onions and rinse them and then cut them into rings.
3. Also, clean the sugar peas, zucchini and mushrooms and cut everything into small pieces.
4. Now heat olive oil in a pan, fry the prepared vegetables in it for about 4 minutes and season everything with salt and pepper.
5. Now add the tomatoes with basil and let it simmer for about 3 minutes.
6. Put in the pieces of fish and cover and let everything simmer for about 5 minutes over low heat.
7. Finally, season it with salt and pepper, cut the chives into fine rolls and sprinkle them over the fish.

BAKED FISH FILLET ON TOMATOES WITH HERBS

10 minutes

30 minutes

2 Servings

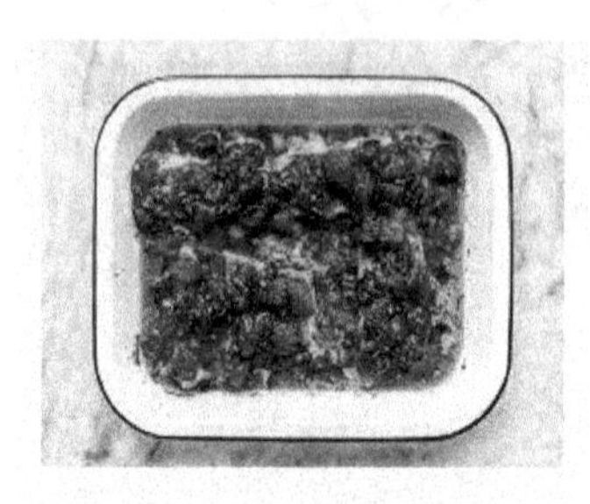

INGREDIENTS

- 350 g lean fish fillet (e.g. pollack, redfish)
- 4 tomatoes
- 2 cloves of garlic
- 4 tbsp sage
- 60 g parmesan cheese
- Salt pepper

COOKING STEPS

1. Rinse off the lean fish fillet, then pat dry and place in a small baking dish.
2. Now season it with salt and pepper, depending on your taste.
3. Next, rinse the beefsteak tomatoes, clean them and cut them into small cubes.
4. Mix the tomatoes with salt and pepper and the crushed cloves of garlic and chopped sage.
5. Spread the mixture over the fish and sprinkle freshly grated parmesan over the top.
6. Now bake everything in the hot oven (200 ° C / fan oven: 180 ° C) for about 15-20 minutes.

ZUCCHINI SALAD WITH COD

10 minutes

40 minutes

1 Servings

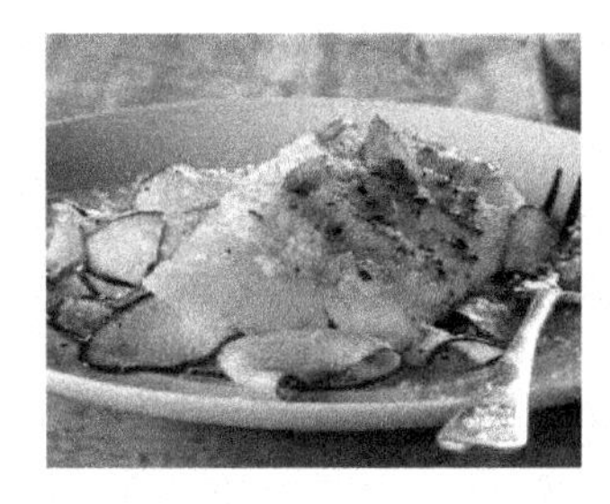

INGREDIENTS

- 280 g zucchini
- 1 tbsp cress
- 100 g lamb's lettuce
- 150 g of cod
- 30 g pecorino (cheese)
- Salt, pepper, chili powder

COOKING STEPS

1. Preheat the oven to 180 ° C. Place the cod in a baking dish and season with salt, pepper and chili flakes.
2. Finally, pour a little more oil over it. Let the whole bake for 25-35 minutes.
3. Wash the zucchini, cut into slices and then place on a baking sheet. Season with salt and pepper and also pour oil over it.
4. These are also put in the oven for about 10 minutes.
5. Wash the lamb's lettuce thoroughly and then mix it with the zucchini.
6. Put the two things on a plate and place the cod on it and then sprinkle with the cheese and cress.

PIKEPERCH FILLET IN MUSTARD AND CREAM SAUCE

10 minutes

30 minutes

1 Servings

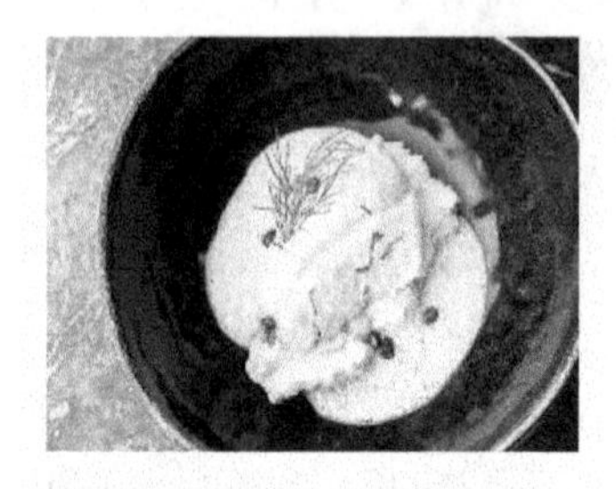

INGREDIENTS

- ½ shallot
- 380 g celeriac
- 150 g pikeperch fillet
- 100 ml of cream
- 50 ml of broth
- 2 tbsp sour cream
- ½ teaspoon lemon juice
- ½ teaspoon mustard
- Salt, pepper, nutmeg

COOKING STEPS

1. Wash the celery and cut into small pieces with the shallot. Heat some oil in a saucepan and add the shallot.
2. Then add the celery and fry briefly. Next, add the broth and simmer for about 15 minutes.
3. The pot is now off the stove and the contents must be mashed with a potato masher.
4. Stir the butter and sour cream into the mixture and season with the spices.
5. Heat the oil in a pan and fry the pikeperch fillet for about 10 minutes.
6. For the sauce, chop the dill and heat the cream in a saucepan.
7. Stir in the mustard, dill and lemon juice and season with spices. Finally serve everything together.

SALMON FILLET WITH CUCUMBER PUMPKIN VEGETABLES

10 minutes

30 minutes

2 Servings

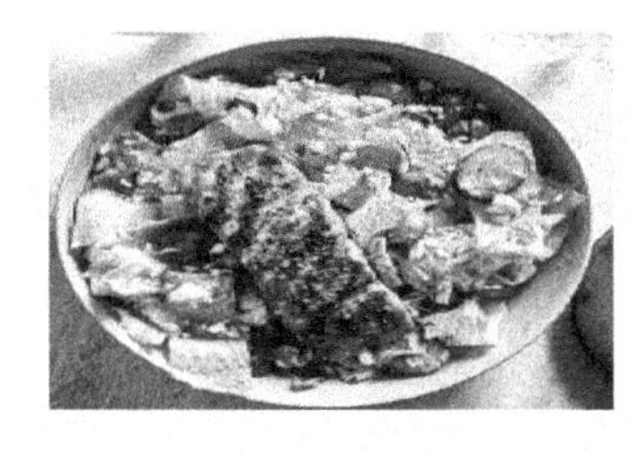

INGREDIENTS

- 400g pumpkin
- 250g cucumber
- 3 shallots
- ½ bunch of dill
- 3 tbsp rapeseed oil
- 100ml broth
- salt and pepper
- 2 teaspoons of honey
- 400g salmon fillet with skin
- 4 tsp sesame seeds
- 4 tbsp fried onions
- 1 tbsp sesame oil

COOKING STEPS

1. Wash and core the pumpkin and dice very finely.
2. Peel, quarter and core the cucumber and cut into half slices.
3. Peel and finely chop shallots. Wash, drain and chop finely the dill.
4. Heat 2 tablespoons of oil in a saucepan and sauté vegetables in it. Deglaze with the broth. Season with salt, pepper and honey. Cover and cook for 15 minutes.
5. Heat 1 tablespoon of oil in a pan and fry the fish on both sides.
6. Toast the sesame without oil until golden brown. Mix the dill and sesame oil into the vegetables.
7. Serve the fish with the pumpkin and cucumber vegetables.
8. Pile the onion and sesame mixture on top of the fish.

COCONUT FISH NOODLES

10 minutes

30 minutes

4 Servings

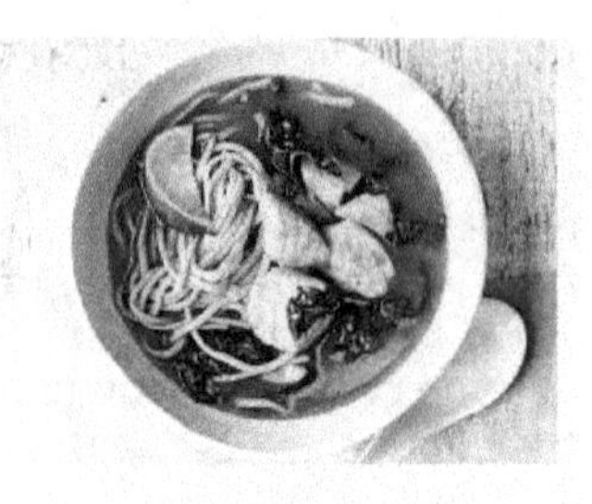

INGREDIENTS

- 140 g onions
- 2 cloves of garlic 500 g carrots
- 250 g zucchini
- 200 g tilapia fillet
- 1 organic lime
- 150 ml classic vegetable stock
- 400 g spaghetti (spelled, whole grain)
- a bit of salt
- 160 ml coconut milk
- 2 tbsp soy sauce
- some cayenne pepper

COOKING STEPS

1. Peel the onions and garlic and cut both into small pieces.
2. Then clean the carrots, peel them with the peeler, halve them lengthways and then cut them into slices.
3. Wash and drain the fish.
4. Wash the lime with hot water and then cut thin slices with the peeler. Then squeeze the limes.
5. In a saucepan, bring the vegetable stock to the boil and add the carrots, onions and garlic. Simmer for 5 minutes with the pot closed.
6. During this time, bring the pasta to the boil in normal salted water.
7. Now add the coconut milk, zucchini and 2/3 of the lime zest to the saucepan.
8. Bring to the boil briefly and then cook for 5 minutes. Add soy sauce.
9. Add the fish to the vegetables after they have been cut into small pieces. Let it cook for 10 minutes.
10. Please keep the pot closed.

11. Drain the spaghetti and serve the sauce with the fish.
12. Don't forget to season everything with the spices.

FISH AND CUCUMBER RAGOUT

10 minutes

50 minutes

4 Servings

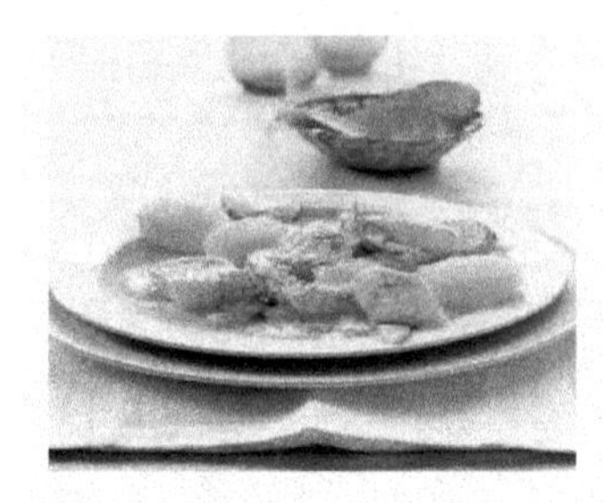

INGREDIENTS

- 300 g pollack fillet (frozen)
- 150 g celeriac
- 2 onions
- a bit of salt
- 3 stalks of dill
- 50 g yogurt (3.5% fat)
- some pepper
- 3 cucumbers
- 2 tbsp olive oil
- 2 teaspoons mustard seeds
- 600 ml classic vegetable stock

COOKING STEPS

1. In the first step, please let the saithe fillet thaw.
2. During this time wash, peel and dice the celery.
3. Peel the onion and also cut it into pieces.
4. Please wash the cucumbers with hot water and then peel them with the peeler. Halve the cucumber lengthways and core it in the middle with a teaspoon.
5. Then cut the cucumber into slices.
6. Heat the oil in a saucepan.
7. Then add the celery, onions and mustard seeds to the pot. Simmer everything for 15 minutes.
8. Then add the cucumber and 100 ml vegetable stock. Bring everything to the boil.
9. Add the rest of the vegetable stock and rice and simmer for 10 minutes.
10. Divide the fish fillet into pieces and season with salt. Place the fish on top of the cucumber vegetables and cook for 15 minutes with the pot closed.
11. Cut the dill into small pieces.

- 250 g long grain rice

12. Mix half of it with the yogurt and add to the ragout. Now serve

FISH STEW WITH VEGETABLES

10 minutes

30 minutes

2 Servings

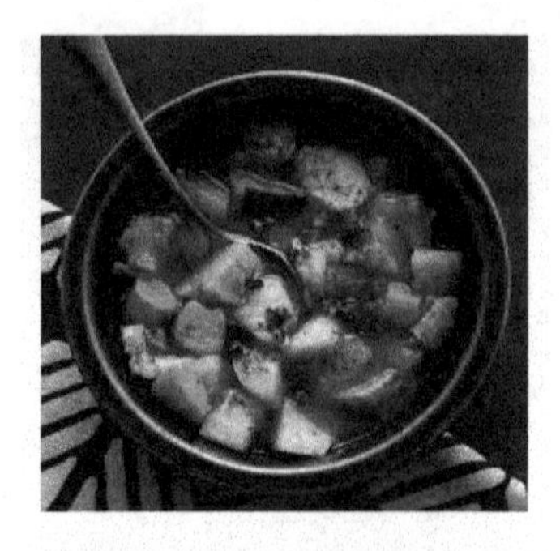

INGREDIENTS

- 2 salmon fillets
- 2 white fish fillets (e.g. pangasius, cod or pollack fillet)
- 1 pack. shrimp
- 3 cans of chunky tomatoes
- 1 bunch of soup greens olive oil
- 2 bay leaves
- 2 cloves of garlic
- 1 medium red onion herbs of Provence
- Chili or cayenne pepper

COOKING STEPS

1. First, sweat the red onions together with the chopped garlic and bay leaves in a little olive oil.
2. Add the very finely chopped soup greens and the lemon zest and sweat them with them until the vegetables have got some color and roasted aromas have developed.
3. If you use sugar, add it now and let the vegetables caramelize for a moment.
4. Now delete everything with a little white wine and let it boil down briefly so that the alcohol initially disappears and only the pure wine aroma remains.
5. If you do not use white wine, add the tomato cans directly, add a little water and let everything boil or boil down briefly as well.
6. Then season it to taste with salt, pepper, herbs of Provence and chili or cayenne pepper.
7. Now add the fish and let it cook for 5 minutes.
8. Then add the prawns and let them steep in the soup.

- Lemon peel, untreated, grated
- possibly white wine
- some sugar
- salt and pepper

QUINOA WITH PRAWNS

5 minutes

15 minutes

2 Servings

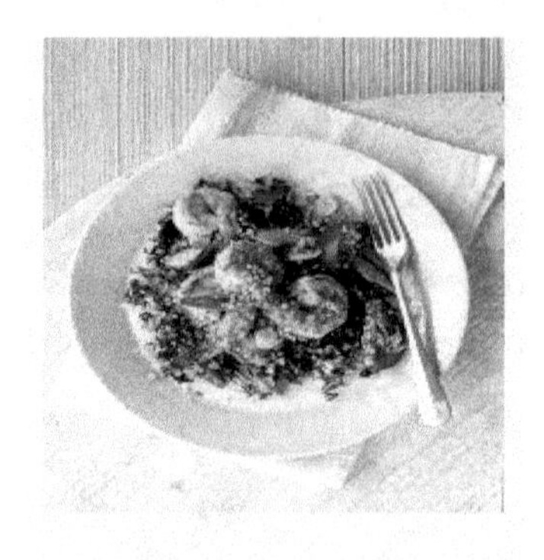

INGREDIENTS

- 1 lemon
- 1 zucchini (small)
- 150 g prawns
- 90 g quinoa
- 800 ml of broth
- 200 ml white wine
- 40 g parmesan
- salt and pepper

COOKING STEPS

1. Put the quinoa in a saucepan with a little oil and let it fry briefly.
2. Deglaze with a little wine and broth. Stir and pour in the broth and wine again and again until nothing is left.
3. Wash the zucchini and cut into small pieces. Wash and dry the prawns as well. Put both ingredients in the pot towards the end.
4. Squeeze the lemon and rub the peel. Now only season to taste with the lemon, salt and pepper.

MONKFISH FILLET IN CURRY SAUCE

10 minutes

15 minutes

4 Servings

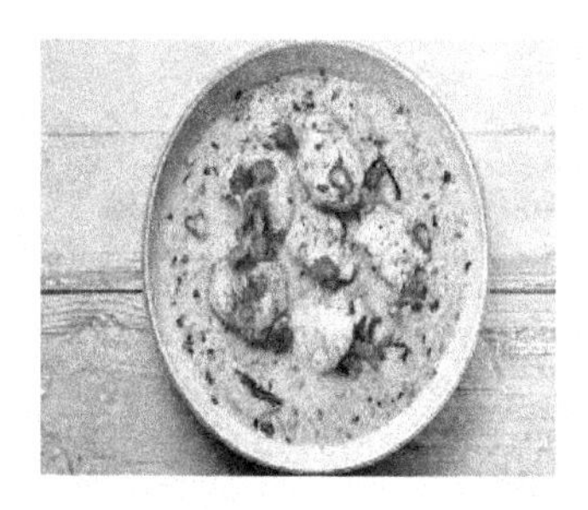

INGREDIENTS

- 4 stalks of coriander
- 6 peppers
- 1 teaspoon mustard seeds
- 600 g monkfish fillet
- 400 ml coconut milk
- 200 ml of broth
- 1 teaspoon lime juice
- 2 tbsp curry powder
- Salt, pepper, chili powder

COOKING STEPS

1. Wash the peppers and cut into small pieces together with the onion.
2. Heat some oil in a pan and add the mustard seeds. Add the stock and coconut milk and season with the curry.
3. Add the peppers and season with salt and chili.
4. Wash the fish and cut into small pieces. Put in the pan and simmer for 5 minutes.
5. Finally, just add the spices to taste and add the lime juice. Scatter coriander on top.

PIKE-PERCH PAN WITH TOMATOES

10 minutes

20 minutes

4 Servings

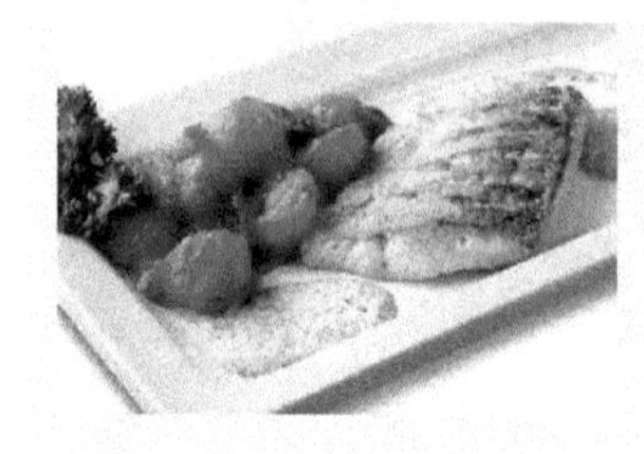

INGREDIENTS

- 2 shallots
- 300 g small tomatoes
- 700 g pikeperch fillet
- a bit of salt
- 3 tbsp wholemeal flour
- 2 tbsp olive oil
- 125 ml white wine
- 200 ml soy cream
- 3 tablespoons of grainy mustard
- some pepper
- 2 stalks of dill

COOKING STEPS

1. Peel the pikeperch fillet and cut into cubes. Please wash the tomatoes and cut them in half.
2. Halve the fish fillet and divide into bite-sized pieces. Then season the fish with salt and pepper and dust with flour. Then shake off the flour.
3. Heat oil in a pan and add the pieces of fish to the pan. Then place the pieces of fish on a plate and add the shallots and tomatoes to the pan.
4. Fry a little and deglaze with white wine.
5. Add the soy cream and taste. Simmer for 2 minutes before stirring the mustard into the sauce and adding the fish to the pan again.
6. Then bring everything to the boil again.
7. Wash and cut the dill and then pour it over the fish as a garnish.

GREEN FISH CURRY

10 minutes

50 minutes

2 Servings

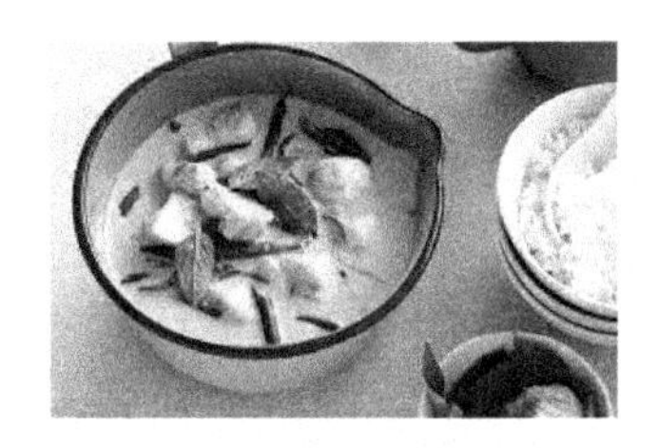

INGREDIENTS

- 1 onion
- 2 cloves of garlic
- 1stick of lemongrass
- 2 tablespoons oil
- 2 teaspoons of green curry paste
- 100 ml coconut milk
- 100 ml coconut water
- 100 ml fish stock
- 1 small Romanesco
- a bit of salt
- 8 cherry tomatoes
- 1 bell pepper
- 2 tbsp Thai fish sauce

COOKING STEPS

1. Peel and finely chop the onion and garlic. Cut the lemongrass into slices.
2. Heat 1 tablespoon of oil in a saucepan and sauté the onion, garlic and lemongrass in it. 3 to 4 minutes are enough. The give curry paste to the pan and saute.
3. Then fill up the coconut milk, coconut water and fish stock. Bring the contents of the pot to a boil and cook for 10 to 15 minutes. Pass the contents through a sieve and keep the broth and the solid contents separately.
4. Clean and chop the romanesco. Then cook the salad in a saucepan for 4 minutes.
5. Then wash the tomatoes and peppers. Cut both into small pieces. Heat the oil in a saucepan or wok and fry the bell pepper with the tomato there.
6. Drain the romanesco and add to the pan.
7. Add the sauce from the first pot and bring to the boil.
8. Add the fish sauce and stir in.

- 300 g tilapia fillet (cichlid)
- some pepper
- 4 stalks of coriander

9. Cut the fish into small pieces and add.
10. Cook for another 10 minutes and add the remaining spices to taste.

WILD GARLIC CRÊPES

5 minutes

10 minutes

4 Servings

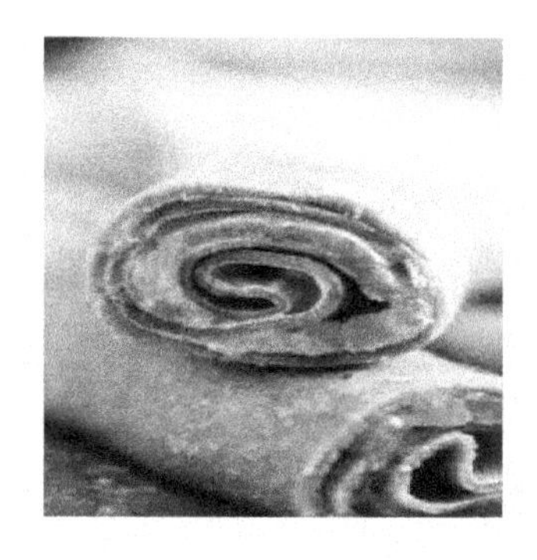

INGREDIENTS

- 250 ml milk
- 125 g flour
- 2 eggs
- 250 g cream cheese
- 150 g sour cream
- ½ lemon
- 50 g wild garlic
- 1 bunch of chives
- 100 g smoked salmon
- salt and pepper

COOKING STEPS

1. Cut the wild garlic and put it in a blender with the milk. Put the eggs in a bowl and add the pureed mass.
2. Then add the flour and mix everything into dough. Then let this dough rest in the refrigerator for 10 minutes.
3. Finely dice the salmon and place in a bowl with the sour cream, lemon juice and zest and cream cheese.
4. Mix everything together and then puree the mixture. Just season with salt and pepper.
5. Take the dough out of the refrigerator and gradually bake it in the pan.
6. Finally, coat the crêpes with the salmon cream and then enjoy.

SMOKED TROUT WITH RED AND YELLOW SALAD

10 minutes

5 minutes

2 Servings

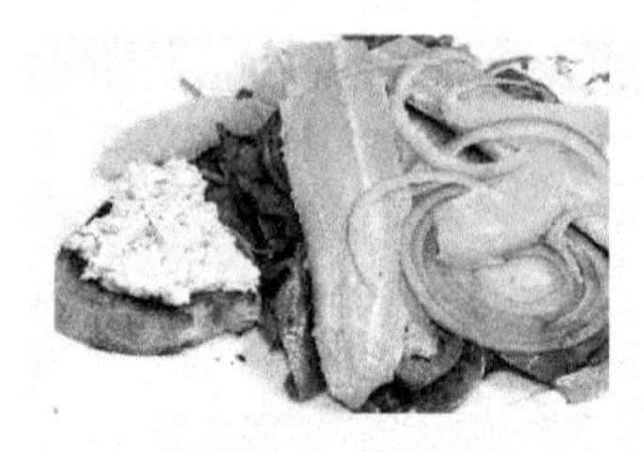

INGREDIENTS

- 125 g smoked trout fillets
- 2 tbsp walnut kernels
- ½ head of red cabbage (approx. 400 g)
- 1 small onion
- 3 tbsp fruit vinegar
- ½ tbsp sunflower oil
- 2 tbsp beetroot sprouts as an alternative to alfalfa sprouts
- 1 oranges
- 35 g dried pitted dates

COOKING STEPS

1. First, toast the nuts in a pan without fat and then remove them. Please clean the red cabbage, wash, quarter and cut out the stalk. Cut the cabbage into fine strips.
2. Peel the onions, cut them in half and cut them into very fine strips.
3. Next, mix the cabbage, onions, vinegar, salt, pepper and oil and knead vigorously with your hands.
4. Then wash the sprouts and let them drain well.
5. Also, wash off the organic orange with hot water, then dry it and rub the peel finely.
6. Peel the two oranges thick enough to completely remove the white skin.
7. Use a sharp knife to cut the fillets out between the separating membranes and squeeze the juice out of the separating membranes.
8. Cut the dates into thin rings and roughly chop the nuts.
9. Now mix the red cabbage salad with the orange peel, fillets and orange

- Salt pepper

juice, dates and nuts and taste everything.

10. Serve the salad with the roughly torn trout fillets and the sprouts.

SALAD WITH CHAR FILLETS

15 minutes

5 minutes

2 Servings

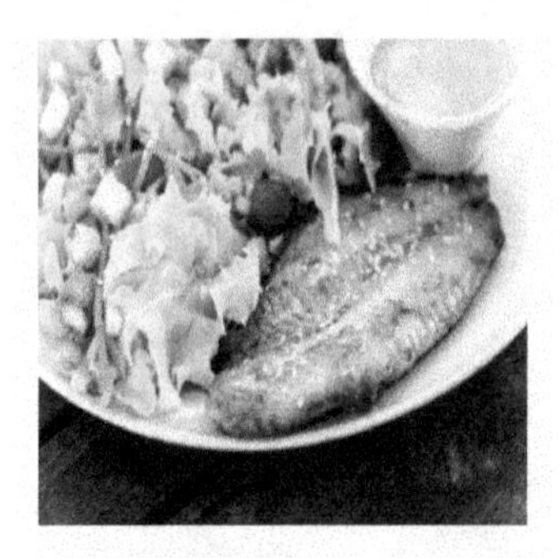

INGREDIENTS

- 1 head Lollo Rosso
- 1 cucumber
- 5 radishes
- 1 clove of garlic
- ½ lemon
- 2 slices of pumpernickel
- 2 tbsp olive oil
- 1 tbsp sesame paste
- 2 char fillets (smoked) salt and pepper

COOKING STEPS

1. Wash the lettuce and radishes and cut them into smaller pieces.
2. Wash half of the cucumber and cut into small pieces.
3. Then mix 1 tablespoon of olive oil, lemon juice, sesame paste, garlic and salt and pepper. Then puree the whole thing.
4. Slice the rest of the cucumber. Cut the pumpernickel into smaller pieces and fry them in a pan to get crispy. Divide the fish into thin strips.
5. Divide the salad into 2 bowls, pour the dressing over it and then spread the pumpernickel and the fish

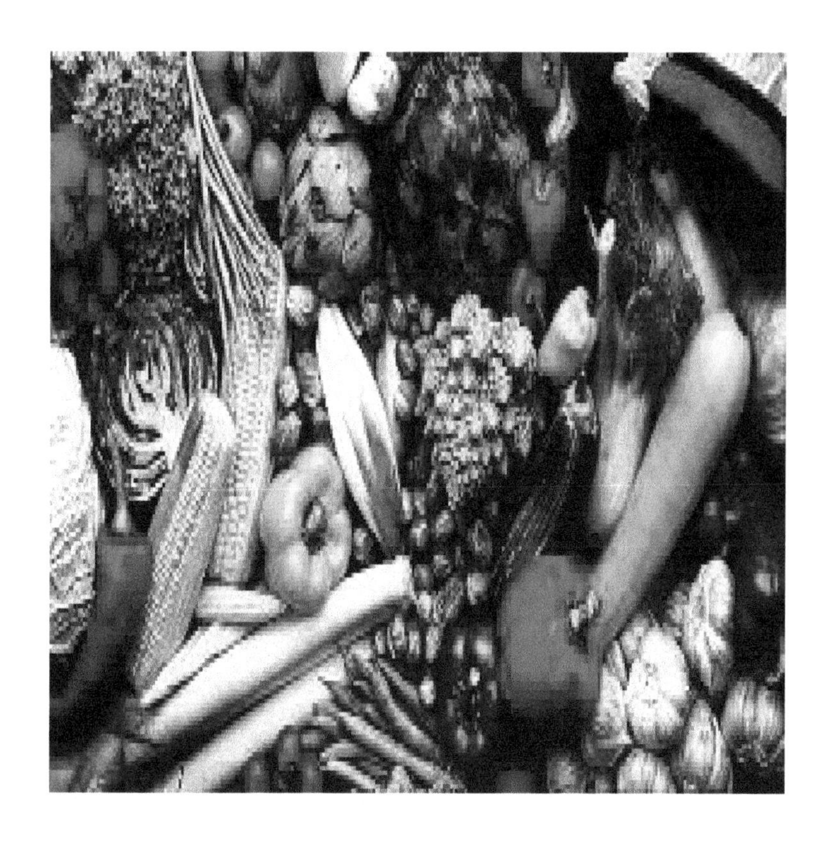

Vegetarian Recipes

WRAPS WITH COUSCOUS AND VEGETABLES

5 minutes

10 minutes

2 Servings

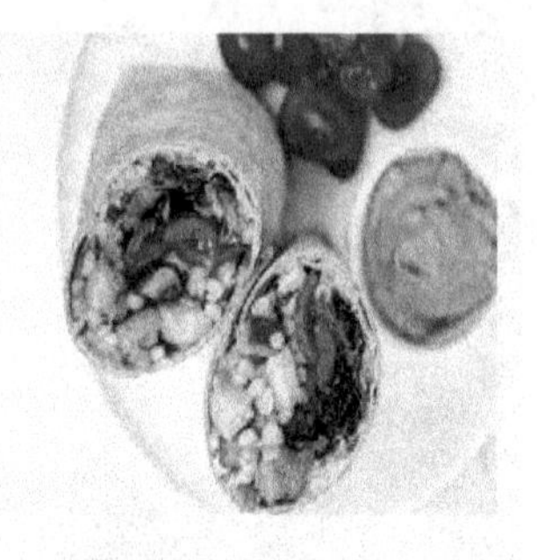

INGREDIENTS

- 250 g zucchini
- 120 g mushrooms
- 160 g paprika
- 2 spring onions
- 120 g tomato paste
- 175 g couscous (cook in advance)
- 200 g natural yogurt salt and pepper
- Chili powder and paprika powder
- Burrito flatbreads

COOKING STEPS

1. The vegetables must be washed and then cut into bite- sized pieces.
2. Then the vegetables come in a pan with oil and must be sautéed.
3. Then the ready-made couscous as well as the spices and tomato paste are added and everything has to be stirred well.
4. Now the yogurt is mixed with the chili and paprika powder.
5. Warm up the cakes according to the instructions on the packet and fill them while they are still warm, as this will prevent them from breaking easily.
6. First comes the yogurt and then comes the couscous and vegetable mixture. Just close it and the meal is ready.

POTATO PANCAKES WITH ZUCCHINI

10 minutes

10 minutes

2 Servings

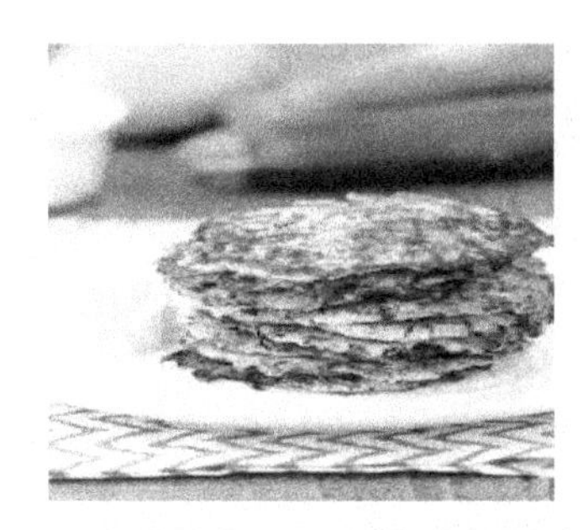

INGREDIENTS

- 3 potatoes
- 3 zucchini
- 1 onion some flour
- 1 egg
- salt and pepper

COOKING STEPS

1. Wash the potatoes and zucchini. Peel the potatoes then grate both the potatoes and the zucchini.
2. Squeeze the grated vegetables in a cloth so that some liquid comes out.
3. Also, cut the onions into small pieces and put everything together in a bowl to make a mass.
4. Shape the mixture into buffers and place them in a pan with a little oil. Fry the buffers on both sides until they turn brown.
5. Then just serve and add a side dish of your choice (e.g. herb quark, applesauce).

CARROT CURRY WITH CHICKPEAS

5 minutes

25 minutes

1 Servings

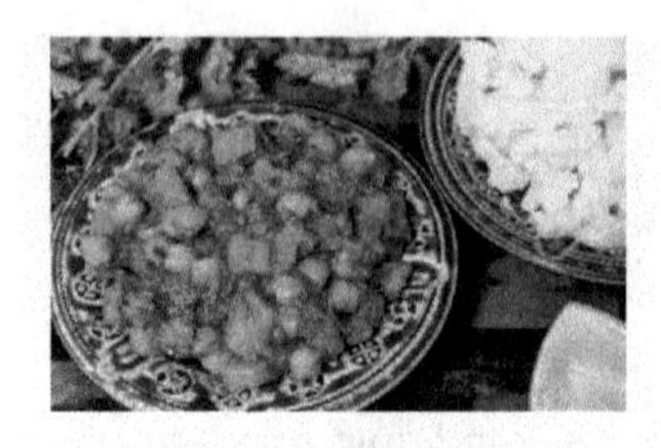

INGREDIENTS

- ½ onion bulb, finely chopped
- ½ pc carrot, cut into cubes
- ½ teaspoon of coconut oil
- ¼ cup of chickpeas
- ½ teaspoon of tomato paste
- 3 tablespoons of light soy cream
- ½ teaspoon of turmeric powder
- ⅛-bunch of fresh coriander
- A pinch of salt, pepper and sweet paprika

COOKING STEPS

1. Sauté the onions and carrots for 5 minutes with coconut oil in a pan.
2. Add the chickpeas, tomato paste, soy cream, turmeric, cilantro and spices.
3. Cook the rice for 10 minutes in boiling water.
4. Serve the konjac rice with the vegetable curry and chickpeas.

BULGUR WITH TOMATOES AND ONIONS

10 minutes

30 minutes

2 Servings

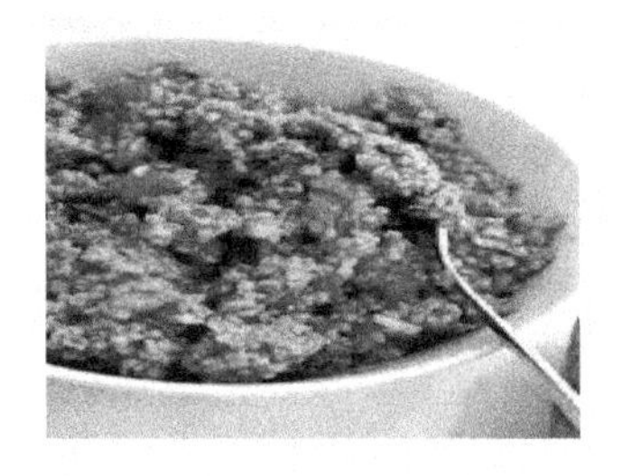

INGREDIENTS

- 750 g onions
- some oil
- 250 g plate lentils
- 500 g bulgur
- 100 ml of olive oil
- 150 g tomatoes
- a bit of salt some pepper

COOKING STEPS

1. In the first step, please boil the lentils in a saucepan with a little salted water.
2. When the lentils are soft, add the bulgur and fill with water until the lentils are covered again.
3. Peel the onions and cut into rings.
4. Then fry in a pan with oil. Wash and chop the tomatoes and add them to the pan as well. Then mix everything well.
5. Add salt and pepper to the bulgur and let it steep.
6. Tip: Salad or bread go perfectly with it.

GREEN SPELLED BALLS

10 minutes

40 minutes

2 Servings

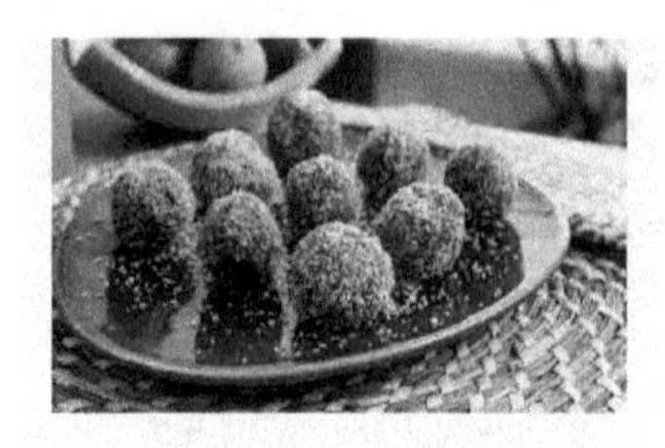

INGREDIENTS

- 100 g green spelled
- 50 g of flaxseed
- 1 red onion
- 50 g spinach leaves
- 2 tablespoons oil
- 1 tbsp mustard
- 1 tbsp sesame mushrooms
- a bit of salt
- some pepper
- 100 ml water, cold
- some oil

COOKING STEPS

1. Pick up a pan and first add the green spelled and flax seeds to roast.
2. Remove the roasted flaxseed and the green spelled and use the mixer to make fine grist.
3. Now peel the onion and cut the spinach into small pieces. Add these two ingredients to the grist.
4. Now add mustard, sesame, water, salt and pepper to the existing mixture. Cover the bowl and let it soak for 10 minutes.
5. Now take a pan and heat the oil. Then shape the mixture into dumplings and fry them.
6. Tip: Go with the salad from our recipe book.

VEGETARIAN VARIETY WITH PEANUT PASTE

10 minutes

15minutes

1 Servings

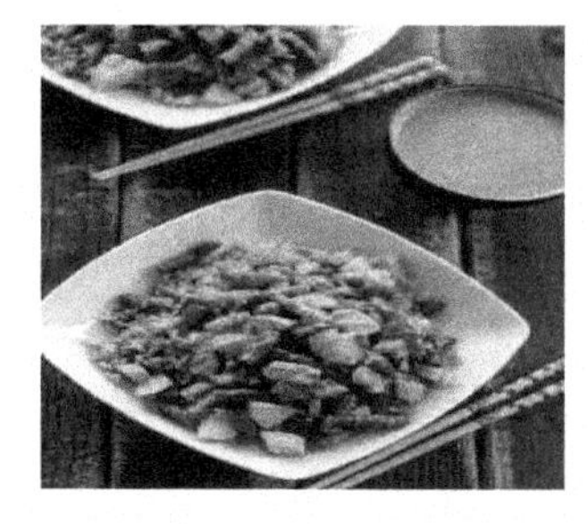

INGREDIENTS

- 1 small onion bulb, thinly sliced
- ¾ cup broccoli, cut into wedges
- 1 pc small carrot, cut into wedges
- ½ pc green pepper, thinly sliced
- 5 mushrooms, cut into wedges
- A pinch of salt, pepper and chili powder
- 2 tablespoons of peanut butter, dairy free

COOKING STEPS

1. Pour a little water into a heated pan and cook the onions until they are transparent.
2. Add the broccoli, carrot, pepper and mushrooms.
3. Cook 10 minutes until tender. (Add water if the pan is too dry). Season the vegetables with a pinch of salt, pepper and chili.
4. For the sauce, mix the peanut butter with the soy sauce, agave syrup and 3 tablespoons of water.
5. To serve, stir in the red cabbage. Garnish the dish with the sauce.

- 2 tbsp. soy sauce, gluten free
- 1 tablespoon of agave syrup (or honey), gluten free
- ¼ cup red cabbage, thinly sliced

AVOCADOS ON TOASTED SPREADS

10 minutes

5 minutes

2 Servings

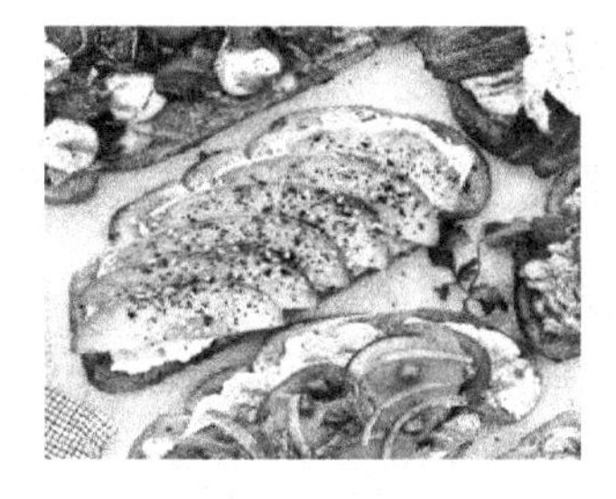

INGREDIENTS

- 2 slice bread, gluten free
- ½ pc small avocado, thinly sliced
- 1 tablespoon of cream cheese
- 1 teaspoon of lemon juice
- Pinch of salt and pepper
- 1 teaspoon of chia seeds for garnish (optional)

COOKING STEPS

1. Lightly toast the slices of bread.
2. Carefully arrange the avocado slices on each slice of bread.
3. Drizzle with lemon juice. Spread the cream cheese.
4. Sprinkle with pepper and salt. Garnish with garnish.

LENTIL SOUP

10 minutes

20 minutes

4 Servings

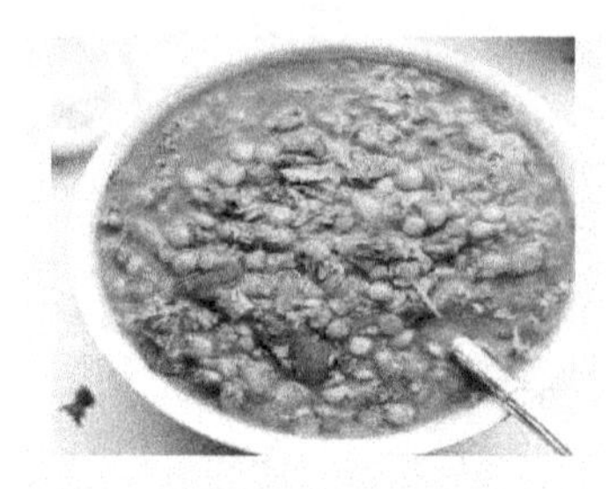

INGREDIENTS

- 1 L vegetable stock
- 200 g lentils (red)
- 2 carrots
- 200 g yogurt
- 2 onions
- Lemon juice
- 2 tbsp butter
- salt and pepper

COOKING STEPS

1. The first thing to do is to cut the carrot and onions into small pieces.
2. These are then put in a saucepan with a little butter and fried for a few minutes.
3. The lentils are also rinsed in a sieve and then put in the pot.
4. Then the vegetable stock is added and the whole thing has to simmer for about 10 minutes with the lid closed.
5. The lentils now need to be mashed.
6. The pot comes off the hot plate and the yogurt and the remaining spices are added and the soup has to be seasoned.

WRAPS WITH COUSCOUS AND VEGETABLES

5 minutes

10 minutes

1 Servings

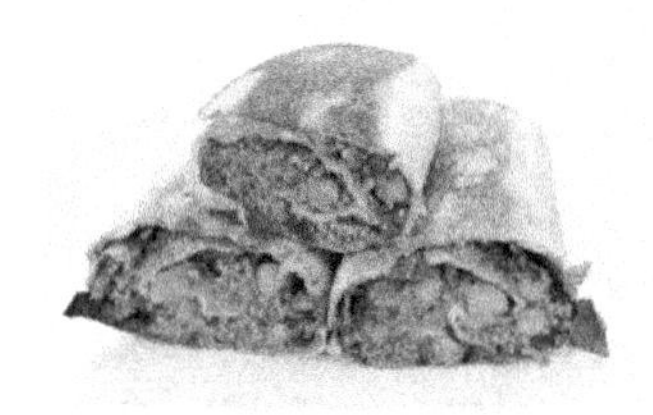

INGREDIENTS

- 250 g zucchini
- 120 g mushrooms
- 160 g paprika
- 2 spring onions
- 120 g tomato paste
- 175 g couscous (cook in advance)
- 200 g natural yogurt salt and pepper
- Chili powder and paprika powder
- Burrito flatbreads

COOKING STEPS

1. The vegetables must be washed and then cut into bite- sized pieces.
2. Then the vegetables come in a pan with oil and must be sautéed.
3. Then the ready-made couscous as well as the spices and tomato paste are added and everything has to be stirred well.
4. Now the yogurt is mixed with the chili and paprika powder.
5. Warm up the cakes according to the instructions on the packet and fill them while they are still warm, as this will prevent them from breaking easily.
6. First comes the yogurt and then comes the couscous and vegetable mixture. Just close it and the meal is ready.

MEDITERRANEAN SPINACH CASSEROLE

10 minutes

20 minutes

4 Servings

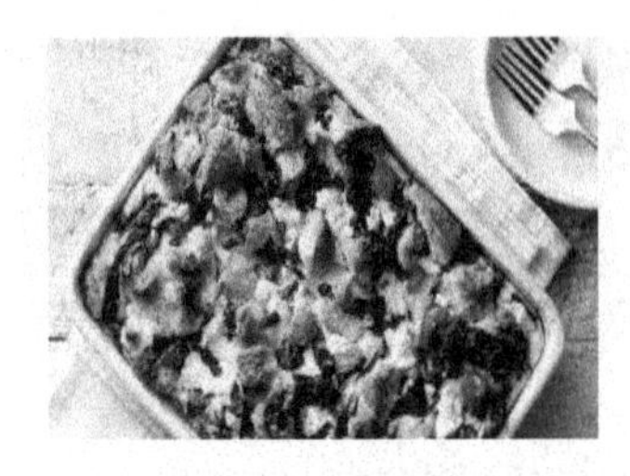

INGREDIENTS

- pounds of fresh baby spinach
- 5 tbsp butter
- tbsp olive oil
- 3 cloves of chopped garlic
- 1 tbsp Italian spices
- ¾ teaspoon salt
- cup of grated parmesan cheese

COOKING STEPS

1. Preheat the oven to 200 degrees (or the highest temperature).
2. Bring five cups of water to a boil in a saucepan and add the spinach for about a minute. Then take it out and drain well.
3. Heat oil and butter in a pan and fry the Italian spices and garlic and season with salt. Cook for about 1 to 2 minutes until the garlic is soft.
4. Put the garlic mixture in a baking dish and spread the oily mixture around the edges of the dish as well.
5. Now add the spinach and sprinkle the spinach with the grated Parmesan.
6. Now put it in the oven for about 10 to 15 minutes.

MUSHROOM CREAM SOUP

10 minutes

20 minutes

2 Servings

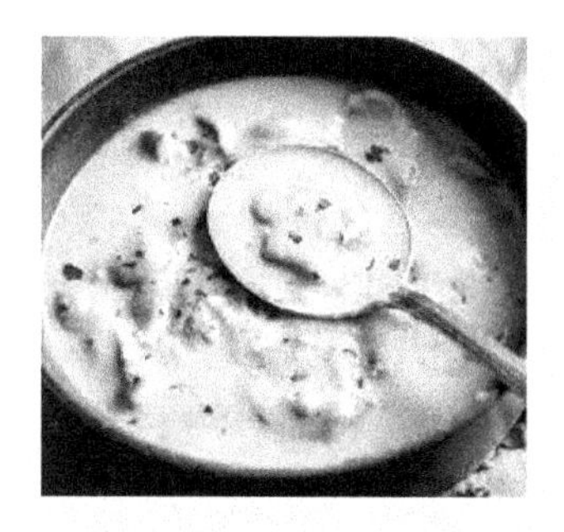

INGREDIENTS

- 4 florets of cauliflower
- 125 g mushrooms
- 1 medium onion
- 200 ml vegetable stock
- 1 tbsp rapeseed oil
- 50 ml milk Salt pepper

COOKING STEPS

1. Cut the cauliflower florets out of the cauliflower head and wash them briefly with water.
2. Please cut the mushrooms into slices and the onion roughly into strips.
3. Now heat the oil, fry the cauliflower florets and the onion in it and let it simmer for about 5 minutes.
4. Now add the mushrooms and fry them.
5. Then take out 2 tablespoons of mushrooms and set them aside.
6. Now pour in the broth and milk and season everything with salt and pepper.
7. Let the soup cook for about 15 minutes and then puree everything.
8. Lastly, taste the soup and garnish with the mushrooms.

NOODLE SOUP

10 minutes | 20 minutes | 2 Servings

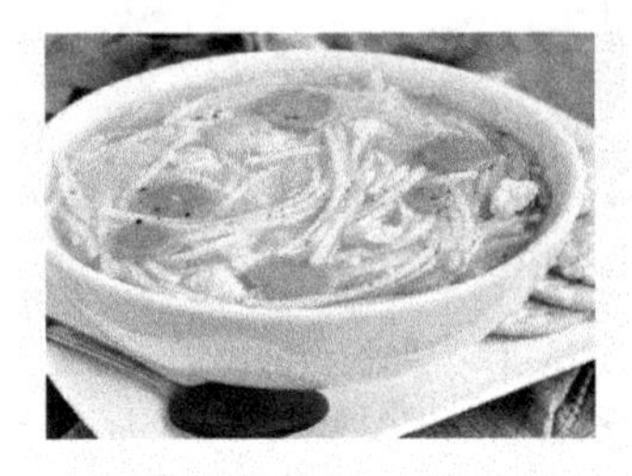

INGREDIENTS

- 1 onion
- 400 g carrots
- 2 stalks of celery
- 150 g frozen peas
- 1 L vegetable stock
- 300 g of soup noodles

COOKING STEPS

1. Please wash and chop the onions, carrots and celery.
2. Then put the prepared vegetables in a saucepan and cook with the vegetable broth.
3. Then add the pasta and peas and cook for another 10 minutes.

BEAN RICE WITH TOFU

10 minutes

40 minutes

2 Servings

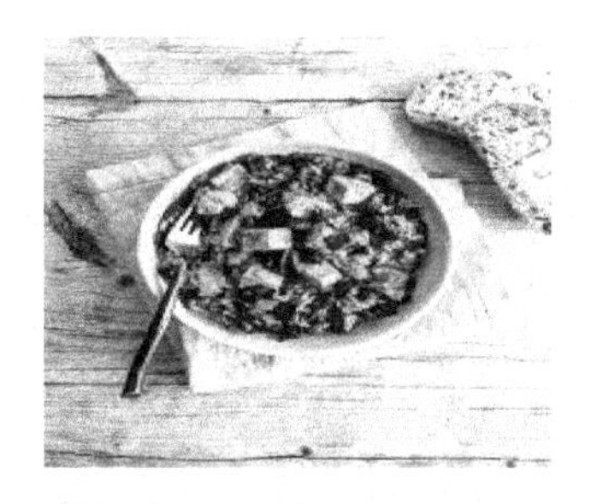

INGREDIENTS

- 175 g dried kidney beans
- 2 cloves of garlic
- 1 onion
- 2 tablespoons oil
- 259 g basmati rice
- 400 ml vegetable stock
- 250 ml coconut milk
- 200 g tofu
- a bit of salt

COOKING STEPS

1. Please take the beans out of the can and let them drain.
2. Peel and chop the garlic and onion. Now sauté these two ingredients in a saucepan.
3. After 5 minutes add the beans and rice and sauté everything briefly.
4. Then add the vegetable stock and milk and bring to the boil.
5. Cook the contents of the pot until the rice is cooked through and the sauce has boiled down.
6. In the meantime, take simply the tofu out of the packaging and season with salt and pepper.
7. Then fry in a non- stick pan with oil. Serve everything together on a plate.

PAPRIKA SAUCE WITH POTATO NOODLES

5 minutes

20 minutes

4 Servings

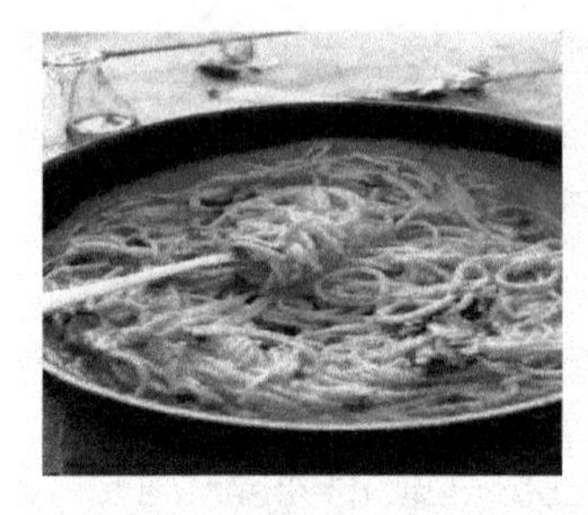

INGREDIENTS

- 500g potato noodles
- 150 ml of cream
- 1 leek
- 2 teaspoons of paprika
- Powder
- 2 teaspoons of smoked paprika powder
- salt and pepper

COOKING STEPS

1. Put the potato noodles in a pan with a little oil and fry them for about 10 minutes.
2. Wash the leek and cut it into rings.
3. The leek is then also in the pan and seared for about 5 minutes.
4. Finally, add the cream and spices. Use more of the spices or other spices, depending on your taste.
5. Let the whole thing cook for about 5 minutes and then serve.

RISOTTO FROM THE OVEN

5 minutes

25 minutes

2 Servings

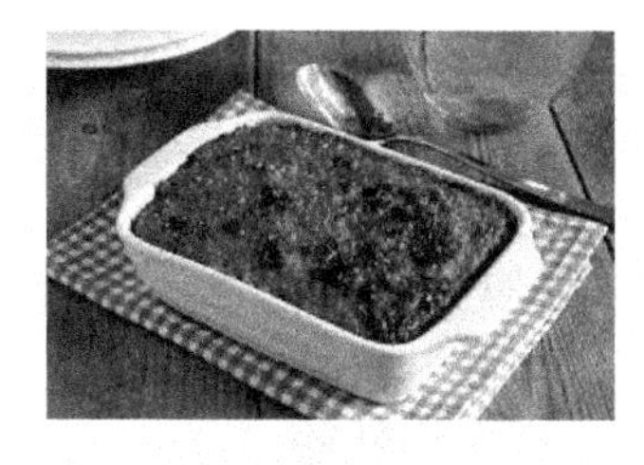

INGREDIENTS

- 300 g pickled peppers
- 1 onion
- 1 clove of garlic
- 2 tbsp parsley
- 275 g rice
- 75 g mozzarella
- 400 g of chunky tomatoes
- 450 ml vegetable stock
- salt and pepper

COOKING STEPS

1. Preheat the oven to 200 ° C top and bottom heat.
2. Cut the onion into small pieces.
3. Put the peppers in a sieve and drain, pat the mozzarella dry with a paper towel and then cut into pieces.
4. Put some oil in a pan and fry the onions for about 6 minutes. Then squeeze the garlic into the pan and cook for another minute.
5. The rice is also in the pan and then 375 ml of stock, the tomatoes and the peppers.
6. The pan must now be put in the oven with the lid on for about 20 minutes.
7. Finally, the mozzarella and the rest of the broth are added and the whole thing has to be seasoned with spices.

PIZZA PIE WITH CHEESE CAULIFLOWER CRUST

5 minutes

30 minutes

2 Servings

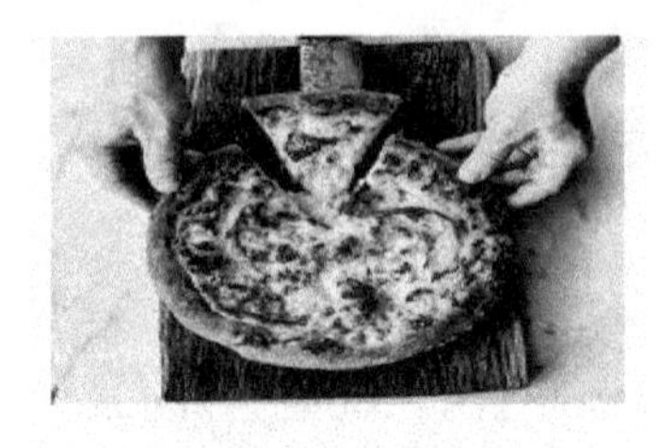

INGREDIENTS

- Cauliflower ½ head, rinsed, chopped, cooked 5 minutes in boiling water and drained
- 2 eggs, beaten
- ⅓-parmesan cheese
- ½ cup cherry tomatoes, washed and cut in half
- 2 tablespoons of organic hemp seed oil
- 1 teaspoon of balsamic vinegar
- 1 ball of mozzarella cheese, crumbled
- ¼ cup basil leaves

COOKING STEPS

1. Swirl the cooked cauliflower in a tea towel to let out as much liquid as possible. (The goal is to get a floury texture.)
2. Add the eggs and cheese. Mix well.
3. Spread the cauliflower paste on a baking sheet lined with parchment paper.
4. Bake for 15 minutes at 400 ° F in your preheated oven.
5. Meanwhile, mix the tomatoes with the hemp oil and balsamic vinegar.
6. Season the mixture with salt and pepper.
7. Remove the pizza dough from the oven. Add the tomato mixture and sprinkle with mozzarella.
8. Return the pan to the oven and continue cooking for 15 minutes.
9. Serve hot and garnish with fresh basil leaves.

SPAGHETTI WITH ASIAN SAUCE

10 minutes

15 minutes

2 Servings

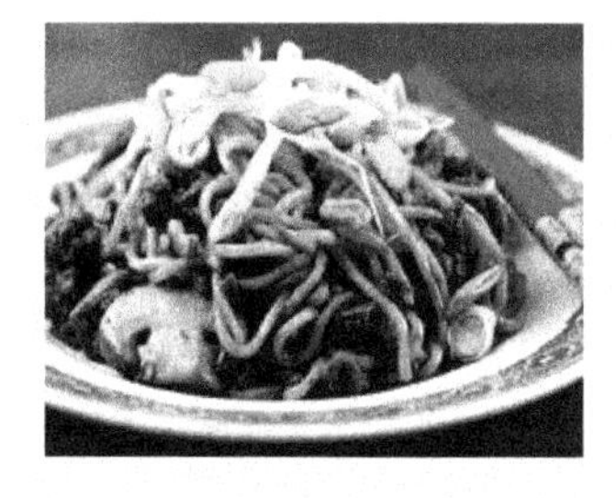

INGREDIENTS

For the sauce:

- 2 tablespoons of soy sauce, gluten free
- 1 teaspoon of hemp oil
- 1 teaspoon of lemon juice
- 1 tablespoon of peanut butter

For the spaghetti:

- ½ onion bulb, diced
- 1 teaspoon of coconut oil
- 1 teaspoon red or green bell pepper, diced

COOKING STEPS

1. Combine all the ingredients for the sauce in a bowl. Put aside.
2. Sauté the onion in the oil and add the peppers, carrots, egg, sauce and spaghetti.
3. Cook 13 minutes, stirring frequently.
4. To serve, garnish with fresh cilantro and peanuts.

- 1 carrot, thinly sliced lengthwise
- 1 egg, beaten
- 5 oz. low-carb spaghetti, rinsed and cooked for 2 minutes in boiling water
- Fresh cilantro and peanuts for garnish

ZUCCHINI GAZPACHO

10 minutes

0 minutes

2 Servings

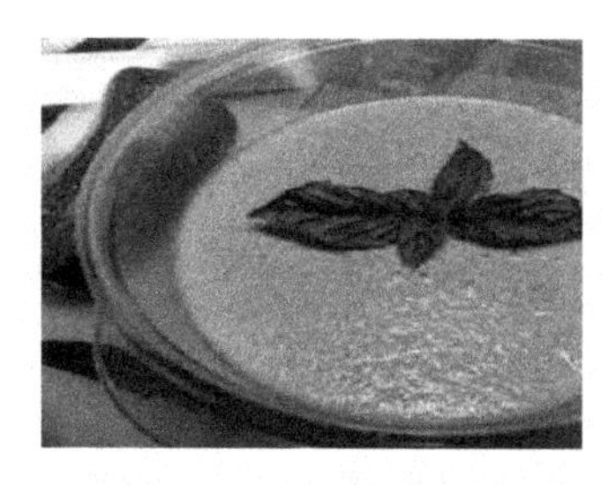

INGREDIENTS

- 4 medium zucchini
- ½ green pepper
- ½ onion
- ½ cucumber
- 1 clove of garlic
- 3 slices of bread without crust
- 2 basil leaves
- vinegar
- olive oil salt
- hard-boiled eggs
- Cherry tomatoes for garnish

COOKING STEPS

1. Soak the bread with a little vinegar.
2. Wash the zucchini well and cut into pieces without peeling them.
3. Put in the blender with pepper, onion, cucumber, garlic clove and basil leaves.
4. Add the bread and whip until it becomes a very fine cream.
5. Add a dash of oil and a little salt, if you like, and then stir everything together
6. Store in the refrigerator so that it is very cold at the time of consumption.
7. To serve, cut the hard-boiled eggs and thinly slice the tomatoes and place a little of both in the bowls with the gazpacho, then pour a fine drizzle of oil on top.

QUICHE WITH PICKLED TOMATOES

10 minutes

40 minutes

2 Servings

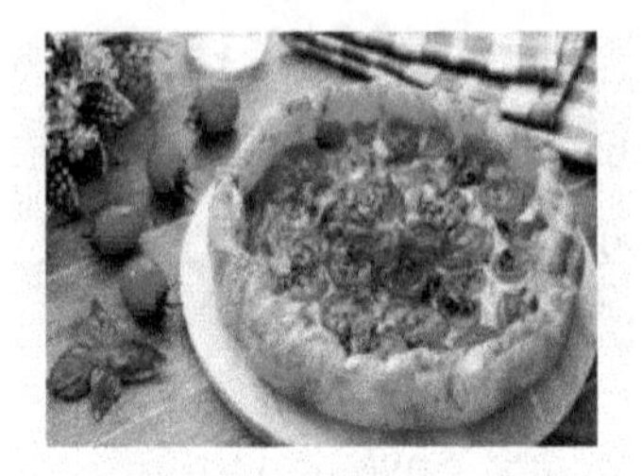

INGREDIENTS

- 100 g ground almonds
- 100 ml of olive oil
- 4 eggs
- 120 g low-fat quark
- 2 green onions
- 1 clove of garlic salt and pepper
- 15 tomatoes in oil
- 200 ml cooking cream
- 2 tbsp rosemary
- 125g whole wheat flour

COOKING STEPS

1. Preheat the oven to 180 degrees and brush a springform pan with oil.
2. Knead the almonds, wholemeal flour, olive oil and low- fat quark into dough. Before kneading, add a little salt and the rosemary.
3. Now peel the onion and garlic. Cut the onion into fine slices and the garlic into fine cubes.
4. Cut the tomatoes into pieces and briefly sweat them and the onion and garlic in a pan.
5. After that, spread these ingredients out on the pre-baked base.
6. Whisk the eggs with the cream, cheese and rosemary.
7. Spread the mixture evenly and bake the quiche in the oven for another 25 minutes.

FRENCH RATATOUILLE SALAD

10 minutes

20 minutes

3 Servings

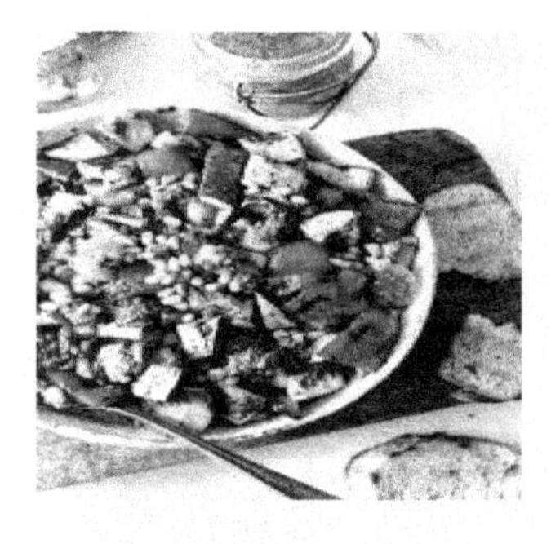

INGREDIENTS

- 3 peppers
- 2 zucchini
- 1 tbsp balsamic vinegar
- 2 red onions
- 20 g parmesan cheese
- 2 cloves of garlic
- 2 sprigs of rosemary
- Salt pepper
- 2 tbsp olive oil
- 300 g tomatoes

COOKING STEPS

1. Preheat the oven to 200 degrees.
2. Wash and clean the peppers and cut them into strips.
3. Wash the zucchini and remove the roots and cut the vegetables into large cubes. Put both in a bowl to mix.
4. Peel off the garlic cloves and press it into the vegetables.
5. Wash the rosemary sprigs, pluck the needles off and chop them up. Mix this with the vegetables with salt, pepper and olive oil and spread everything on a baking sheet. Now put in the oven for 15 minutes.
6. Wash the tomatoes and cut them into wedges.
7. Wash the basil and pluck the leaves and chop them up.
8. Take the vegetables out of the oven and place them in a bowl and add the tomatoes, basil and balsamic vinegar. Slice the parmesan cheese over it.

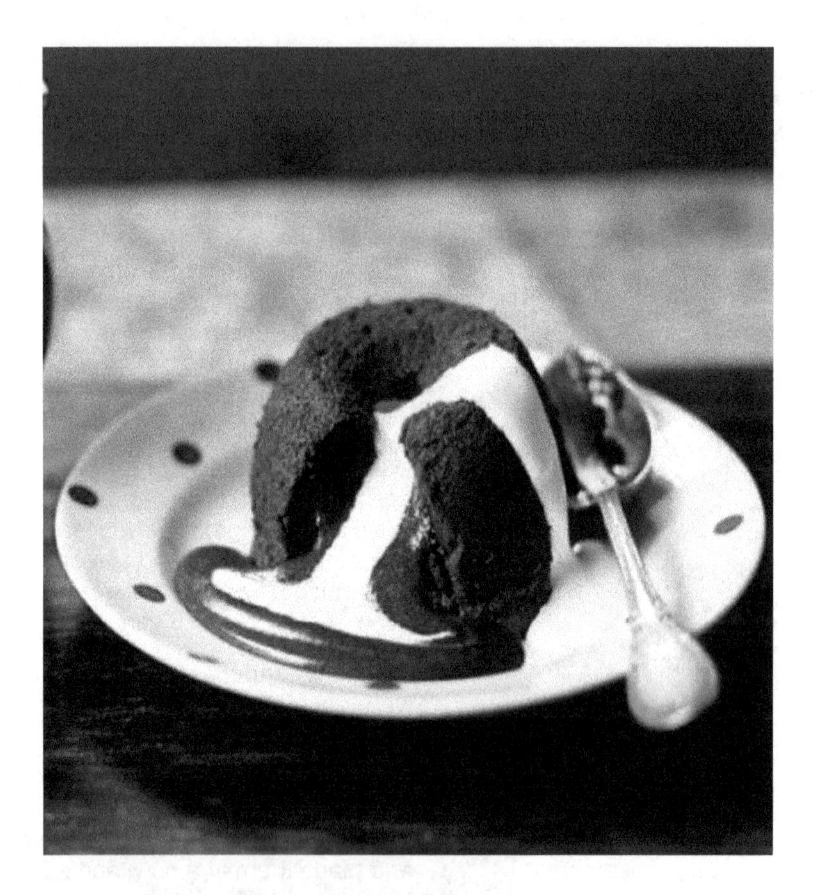

Dessert Recipes

APPLE PIE WITH HONEY

15 minutes

40 minutes

8 Servings

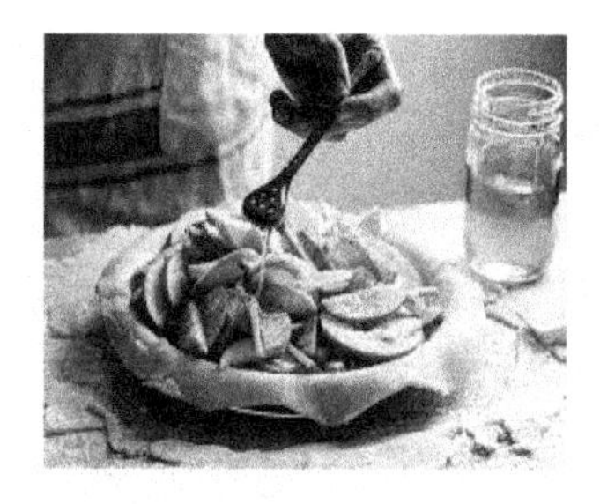

INGREDIENTS

- 90 g whole wheat flour
- 90 g wheat flour
- 90 g butter
- 280 g applesauce
- 3 apples
- 3 eggs
- 5 tbsp honey
- 2 tbsp ground almonds Brown sugar

COOKING STEPS

1. Preheat the oven to 190 ° C.
2. Put the flour in a bowl. Add the butter in smaller slices and then knead until the mixture becomes crumbly.
3. Beat and separate the eggs. Mix one egg yolk with 2 tablespoons of water and then add to the flour. Process into a soft lump and add a little more water if necessary.
4. Flour lightly the work surface and roll out the dough on top. Then put this in a cake pan.
5. Mix the applesauce with honey and the 2 other egg yolks. Add the almonds and mix everything well. Then pour this mixture onto the dough in the mold.
6. Wash the apples and cut into thin wedges. Place these on top of the dough and sprinkle with brown sugar. Put the cake in the oven for 40 minutes. In the end, just garnish with honey.

SWEET STRAWBERRIES COATED WITH CHOCOLATE

3 hours

0 minutes

8 Servings

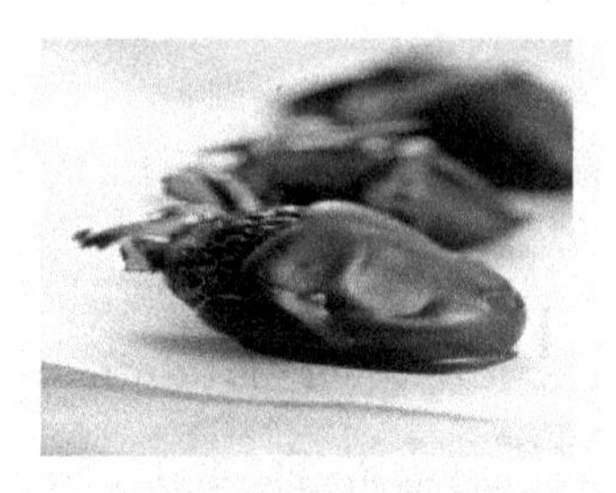

INGREDIENTS

- cups of melted chocolate chips, dairy free
- 2 tablespoons of coconut oil
- 16 fresh strawberries, with stems

COOKING STEPS

1. Combine melted chocolate and coconut oil in a medium bowl.
2. Mix well until well combined.
3. Pour the chocolate mixture into each mold of an ice cube tray.
4. Garnish each with a strawberry, stem side up. Pour the rest of the chocolate mixture over the strawberries.
5. Freeze at least 3 hours until the chocolate hardens.

AMBROSIAL AVOCADO PUREE PUDDING

5 minutes

0 minutes

3 Servings

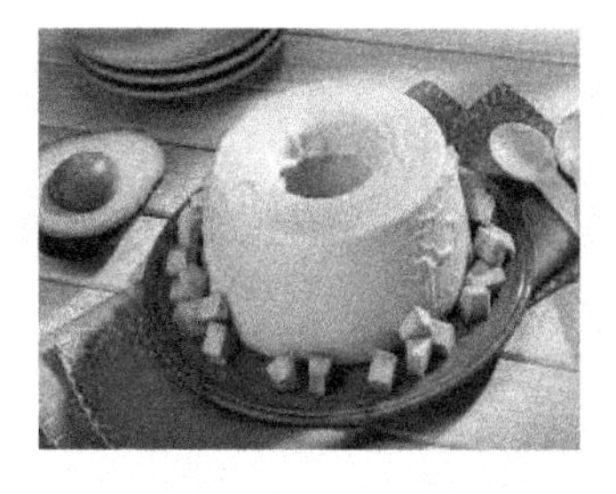

INGREDIENTS

- 2 ripe Hass avocados, peeled, pitted and cut into pieces
- 2 teaspoons of organic vanilla extract
- 80 drops of liquid sweetener
- 1 can (113.5 oz) organic coconut milk
- 1 tablespoon of organic lime juice

COOKING STEPS

1. Combine all the ingredients in a blender. Blend to a smooth, velvety consistency.
2. Pour the mixture equally into three glasses.
3. Refrigerate before serving.

CHOCOLATE COOKIES

25 minutes

25 minutes

4 Servings

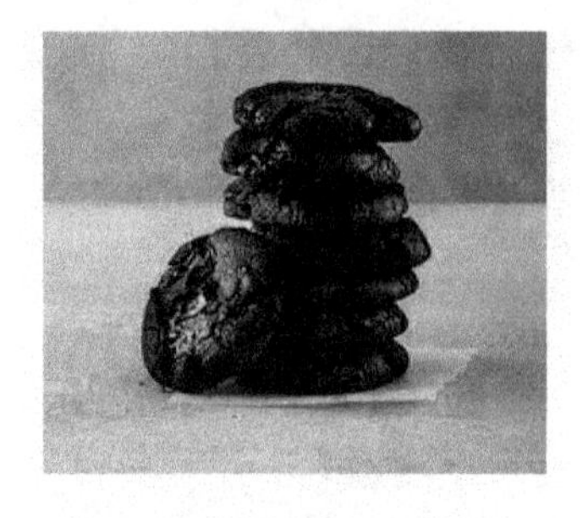

INGREDIENTS

- 130g cocoa powder, unsweetened and de-oiled
- 120g soft butter
- 500g erythritol
- 8 eggs
- 200g almond flour
- 100g flour
- 4 teaspoons of baking powder

COOKING STEPS

1. Preheat the oven to 180 degrees.
2. Work the cocoa powder into a mass in hot water. Mix the butter with erythritol, add the eggs and stir until frothy.
3. Add the flour, almond flour, baking powder and cocoa mass to the butter mass and stir everything well.
4. Line a baking sheet with parchment paper. Shape the dough into small cookies and spread them on the tray.
5. Bake the cookies in the oven for 15 minutes.

RASPBERRY MUFFINS

10 minutes

35 minutes

8 Servings

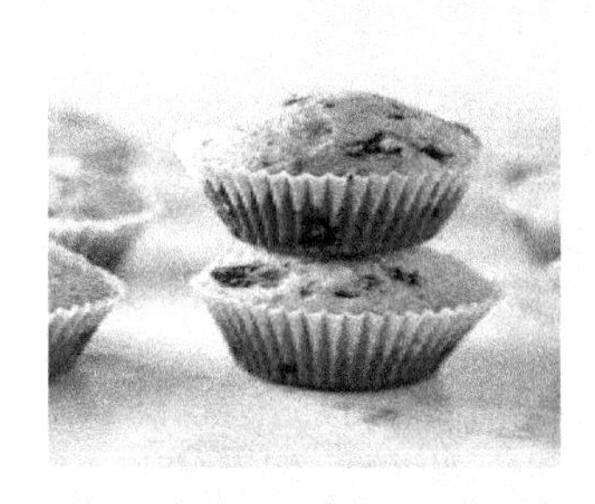

INGREDIENTS

- 200g raspberries
- 150g xylitol
- 100g butter
- 80g almonds, ground
- 80g natural yogurt
- 40g almond flour
- 40g sour cream
- 3 eggs
- 1 pinch of salt
- 1 teaspoon guar gum
- ½ teaspoon baking powder

COOKING STEPS

1. Separate the eggs and beat the egg whites with a pinch of salt to form egg whites.
2. Melt 80 g butter and mix with the egg yolk.
3. Gradually add the guar gum, almond flour, almonds, 70 g xylitol and yoghurt.
4. Mix all ingredients into even dough.
5. Now fold in the egg whites and 150 g raspberries.
6. Pour the batter into muffin cups.
7. Bake at 170 ° C for 20 minutes.
8. In the meantime, prepare the cast.
9. Mix 50 g raspberries with 70 g xylitol, 20 g butter and cream and puree finely.
10. Chill for at least an hour.
11. After cooling, spread the raspberry glaze over the raspberry muffins.

GRAPEFRUIT MOUSSE

20 minutes

2 hours 40 minutes

4 Servings

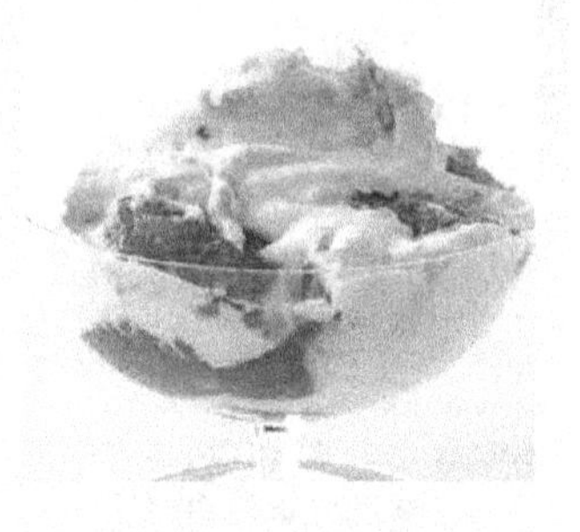

INGREDIENTS

- 200 g whipped cream
- 125 g low-fat quark
- 3 eggs
- 2 grapefruits
- 1 lemon
- 2 tbsp honey
- Gelatin substitute

COOKING STEPS

1. Peel 1 grapefruit, removing the white skin. Then detach the columns and prepare them.
2. Wash the lemon with hot water and rub a little of the peel. Squeeze the second grapefruit and lemon. Soak the gelatin substitute in cold water.
3. Mix the quark with the honey and add the juice of both fruits.
4. Whip the cream until stiff and then stir into the quark.
5. Then stir the gelatin substitute into the cream and place in the refrigerator for 10 minutes.
6. Meanwhile, break the eggs and separate the egg white and yolk. Beat the egg white until stiff and then fold it into the cream.
7. Chill the mousse in glasses for 2 ½ hours. After this time, turn it out onto a plate and serve.

COCONUT BALLS

10 minutes

0 minutes

20 Servings

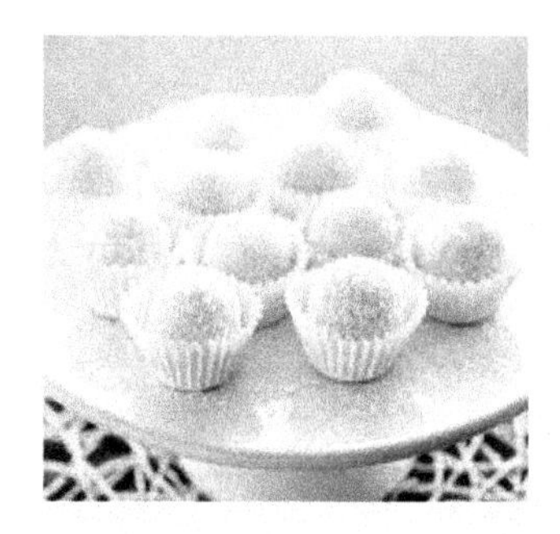

INGREDIENTS

- 80 g desiccated coconut
- 1 can of coconut milk
- 3 tbsp maple syrup
- 20 almonds

COOKING STEPS

1. Skim off the coconut cream and set aside the coconut water.
2. Mix the cream with the maple syrup.
3. Shape the resulting mass into small balls and press one almond per ball into the middle.
4. Prepare the desiccated coconut and roll the balls in them.
5. Then put the finished balls in the refrigerator.

CHOCOLATE CREAM

10 minutes

2 hours

12 Servings

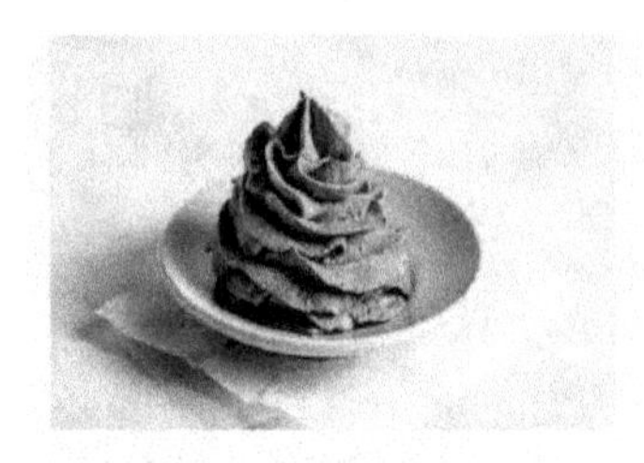

INGREDIENTS

- 300 g vegan dark chocolate
- 150 g xylitol
- 12 blackberries
- 3 packets of cream stabilizer
- 3 pinches of salt
- 3 pinches of cinnamon
- 1 vanilla pod
- 900 ml soy cream
- 30 ml currant liqueur

COOKING STEPS

1. Scrape the pulp from the vanilla pod.
2. In a saucepan, heat the 450 ml soy cream with the pulp of the vanilla pods, the pods, currant liqueur, salt, xylitol and cinnamon. Heat a little more quickly.
3. Add the chopped chocolate and fold it in. Let this melt and then cool everything down to room temperature.
4. Now mix the rest of the soy cream with the cream stiffener and beat it until stiff.
5. Lift the soy cream into the cooled chocolate mixture and fill the dessert bowls with it.
6. These have to cool down for at least 5 hours.

TAPIOCA PUDDING

10 minutes

1 hour

4 Servings

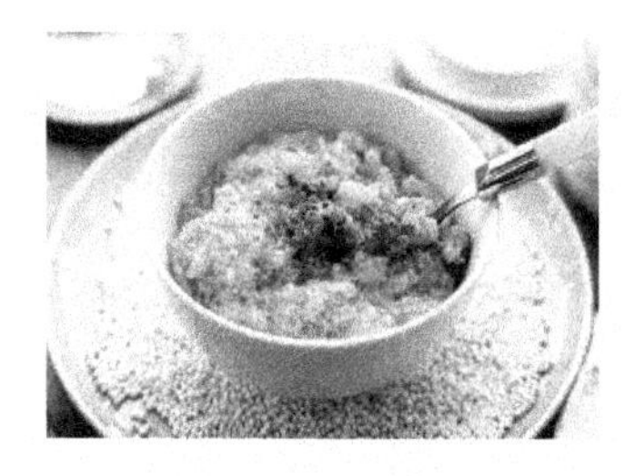

INGREDIENTS

- 40 g tapioca
- 4 peaches
- 3 tbsp xylitol
- 1 tbsp cinnamon
- 300 ml coconut milk
- 200 ml soy cream
- 60 ml sparkling wine

COOKING STEPS

1. Soak the tapioca in hot water for 10 minutes.
2. Then boil the soy cream (100 ml) with xylitol and coconut milk in a saucepan.
3. Then mix in the tapioca pearls and let everything cook on low heat for 20 minutes, stirring constantly.
4. Then let the mixture cool down.
5. Cut the pitted peaches in half. Dust the fruits with cinnamon and grill them on the grill or grill pan for 10 minutes.
6. Dice half of the peaches and mix them with sparkling wine and divide them into four dessert glasses.
7. Then add the pudding.

CREME BRULEE

10 minutes

1 hour

2 Servings

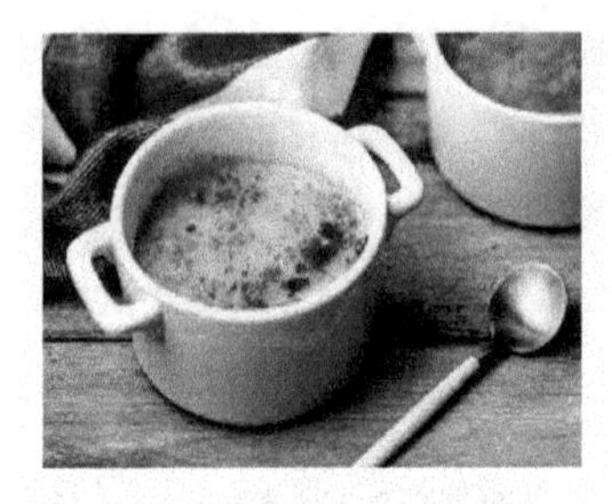

INGREDIENTS

- 30 g cornstarch
- 2 vanilla pods
- 400 ml coconut milk
- 250 ml soy cream
- 10 tbsp erythritol
- 2 tbsp coconut blossom sugar
- turmeric

COOKING STEPS

1. Mix the 3 tablespoons of soy cream with the cornstarch.
2. Heat the rest of the soy cream with the 1 pinch of turmeric, 4 tablespoons of erythritol and the coconut milk.
3. Now mix in the prepared cornstarch and let it boil down over a low heat.
4. Fill the dessert glasses with the cream and chill for 3 hours.
5. Finally, mix the erythritol with the coconut blossom sugar and spread it over the cooled cream.
6. Caramelize with a bunsen burner.

HEALTHY BANANA CAKE

5 minutes

5 minutes

1 Servings

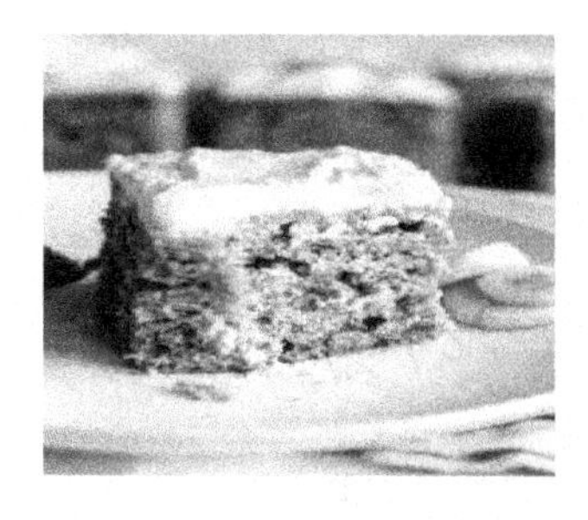

INGREDIENTS

- 35 g spelled flour
- 50 ml soy milk
- 1 banana
- ½ teaspoon cinnamon

COOKING STEPS

1. Peel and mash the banana. Then add the milk and stir in.
2. Add the flour and cinnamon and stir again.
3. Cover and place in the microwave at 200 watts for 2 minutes.

APPLE MILK RICE

10 minutes

15 minutes

1 Servings

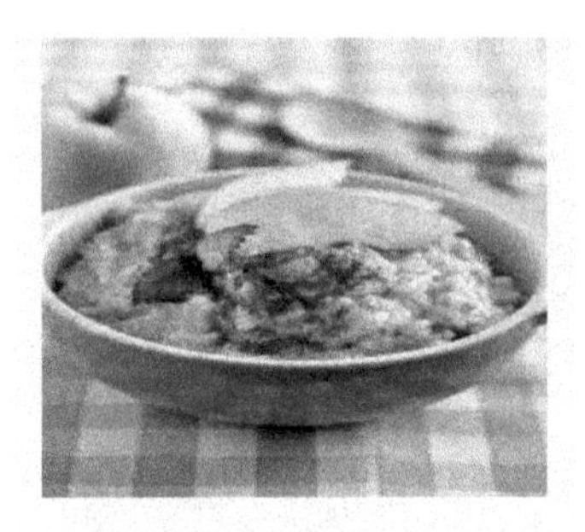

INGREDIENTS

- 25 g protein powder
- 7 tbsp oatmeal
- 1 tbsp sugar
- 185 ml of water
- 1 apple
- 1 pinch of cinnamon

COOKING STEPS

1. Boil the oatmeal in the water until soft.
2. Add the egg white powder and stir until the consistency resembles that of rice pudding and then stir in the sugar.
3. Peel and cut the apple. Stir in half and heat the other half in the microwave.
4. Put the rice pudding in a bowl and garnish with the apple and cinnamon.

BUTTER BALL BOMBS

60 minutes

0 minutes

10 Servings

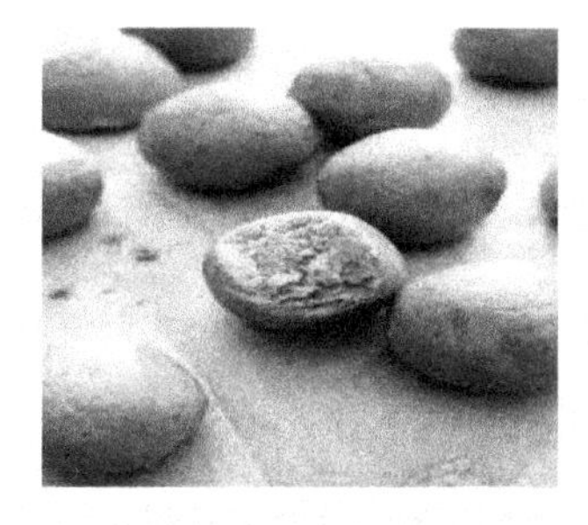

INGREDIENTS

- 8 tbsp (1 stick) butter, softened at room temperature
- ⅓ cup Sweetener
- ½ teaspoon. pure vanilla extract
- ½ teaspoon. kosher salt
- 2 cups of almond flour
- ⅔ cup unsweetened, dairy-free dark chocolate chips

COOKING STEPS

1. Use your hand mixer and beat the butter in a large bowl until light and fluffy.
2. Add the vanilla extract, sweetener and salt. Beat again until completely combined.
3. Gradually add almond flour, beating continuously until no dry portions remain.
4. Add the chocolate chips.
5. Cover the bowl with plastic wrap and refrigerate for 20 minutes until it is slightly firm.
6. Using a small spoon, scoop the dough to form small balls.

MANGO PASSION FRUIT SLICES

40 minutes

60 minutes

20 Servings

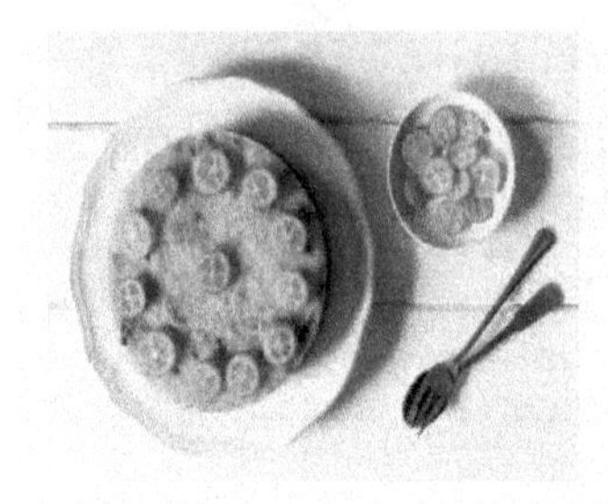

INGREDIENTS

- 500ml whipped cream
- 200g cream cheese
- 130g xylitol
- 125ml mango and passion fruit smoothie
- 100g almond flour
- 6 eggs
- 1 mango
- 4 tbsp yogurt
- 3 tbsp lemon juice
- 3 teaspoons of guar gum
- 1 teaspoon Baking powder

COOKING STEPS

1. Preheat oven to 180 degrees.
2. Beat and separate eggs.
3. Beat the egg whites into egg whites.
4. Put egg yolks, yoghurt, 100g xylitol, almond flour, vanilla flavor, rum flavor, baking powder and guar gum in a bowl and process to a homogeneous mass.
5. Lift the egg whites into the batter.
6. Line the baking sheet with parchment paper and distribute the dough on the sheet. Bake in the oven for 15 minutes.
7. In the meantime, whip the cream until stiff.
8. Add the cream cheese, remaining xylitol and lemon juice to the cream and whisk everything together well.
9. Spread on the cooled dough and set aside.
10. Peel and core the mango and finely puree the pulp in a blender.
11. Add gradually the smoothie and guar gum and then cover and let rest for 30 minutes.

- 1 teaspoon rum flavor
- ½ teaspoon vanilla flavor

12. Now spread on the cake and chill for at least three hours.

STRAWBERRY CAKE

10 minutes

50 minutes

12 Servings

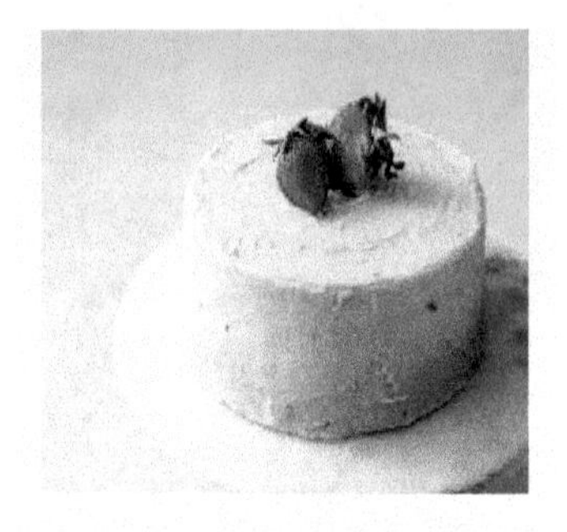

INGREDIENTS

- 750g strawberries
- 250ml water
- 5 eggs
- 2 sheets of gelatin
- 1 vanilla pod
- 5 tbsp xylitol
- 4 tbsp mineral water
- 3 tbsp soy flour
- 1 tbsp lemon juice
- 1 teaspoon Baking powder

COOKING STEPS

1. Preheat oven to 180 degrees.
2. Separate eggs and beat egg whites in a bowl.
3. Halve the vanilla pod and scrape out. Mix the pulp with the egg yolk, baking powder, 4 tablespoons xylitol and mineral water. Add gradually soy flour and continue to stir. Now carefully fold in the egg whites.
4. Pour the dough into a parchment-lined mold.
5. Put the form in the preheated oven and bake for 40 minutes.
6. In the meantime, wash, clean and quarter the strawberries. Spread the strawberries on the cooled base.
7. Soak the gelatine in cold water. Remove and squeeze out after a minute.
8. Heat 250ml water with lemon juice and 1 tablespoon xylitol. Add the soaked gelatine and let it dissolve completely.
9. Immediately distribute the gelatine icing evenly over the strawberry cake.

10. If you want, you can chill the cake for an hour or two before serving.

FROZEN YOGURT

10 minutes

0 minutes

2 Servings

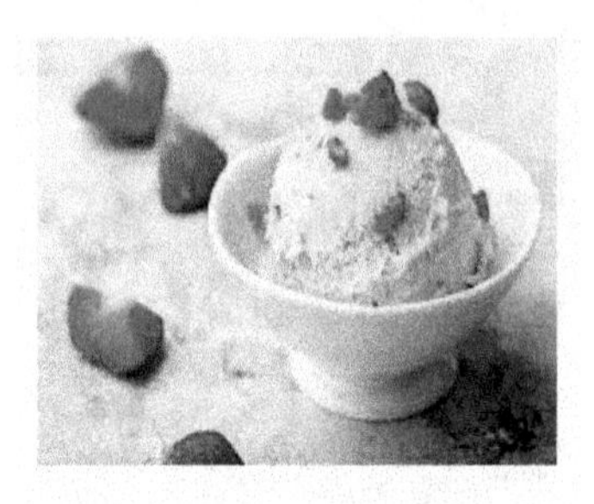

INGREDIENTS

- 500 g quark
- 200 g frozen raspberries
- 2 tbsp sugar

COOKING STEPS

1. Puree the raspberries with a powerful hand mixer.
2. First add half of the quark and puree. Then add the other half and mix again.
3. Divide the yogurt into bowls and either serve immediately or freeze.
4. The chocolate can be melted at will or in pieces as a garnish.

ALMOND BARS

10 minutes

20 minutes

6 Servings

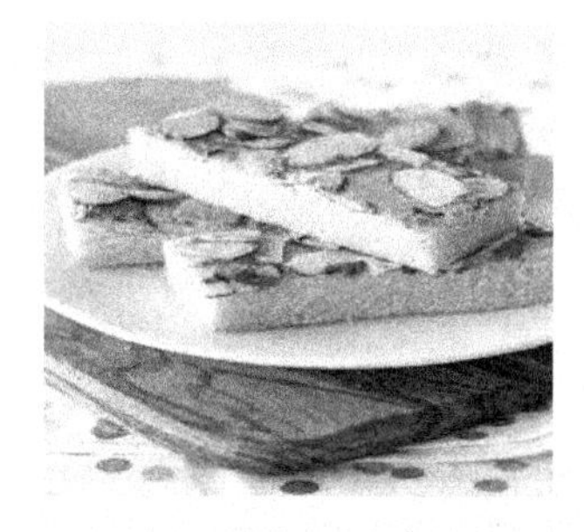

INGREDIENTS

- 1 ¼ cup Almond flour
- ¼ cup Coconut flour
- ½ cup Coconut oil
- 2 tbsp. Almond butter
- ¼ tsp. Salt
- 3 tbsp. Swerve
- 1 tsp. Vanilla extract
- 2 Eggs
- 1 cup Water

COOKING STEPS

1. Place the trivet in the IP and add 1-cup water at the bottom of the stainless steel insert.
2. Combine the ingredients in a food processor and process until sandy texture.
3. Line a small baking pan with some parchment paper and add the dough. Press well with the palm of your hands and gently place in your Instant Pot.
4. Cover with some parchment paper and seal the lid.
5. Press Manual and cook for 15 minutes on High.
6. Release pressure naturally and open the lid.
7. Carefully remove and chill.
8. Slice into 6 bars and refrigerate for 1 hour before serving.

VANILLA CUPCAKES WITH FROSTING

10 minutes

30 minutes

8 Servings

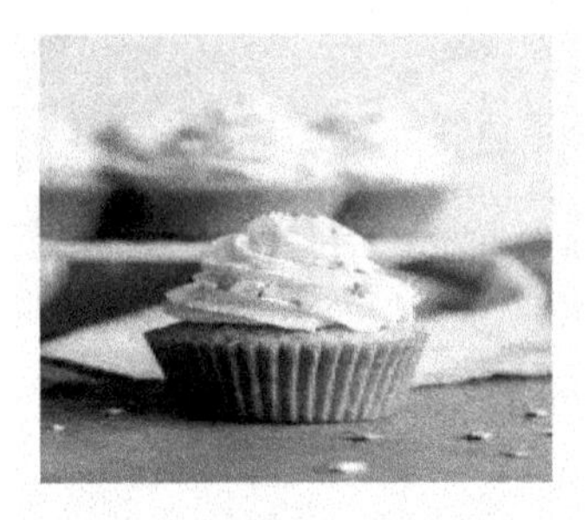

INGREDIENTS

- ½ cup, Butter
- 3 Eggs
- 1 ½ cup Almond flour
- ½ cup
- 2 tsp. Vanilla extract divided in half
- 1 ½ tsp. Baking powder
- 1 cup Cream cheese
- ¼ cup Whipping cream
- 3 tbsp. Powdered erythritol

COOKING STEPS

1. Combine almond flour and swerve in a bowl.
2. Add butter, eggs, and 1 tsp. vanilla extract. Use a hand mixer and beat on high speed until mixed.
3. Transfer the mixture to 8 silicon muffin cups and set aside.
4. Place the trivet at the bottom of the stainless steel insert.
5. Add 1 cup water and gently place the muffin cups on top. Cover loosely with aluminum foil and seal the lid.
6. Press Manual and cook for 15 minutes on High.
7. Do a quick release when done and carefully remove the cups and transfer to a wire rack to cool.
8. Meanwhile, combine the remaining ingredients in a bowl. Beat on high speed until light and fluffy.
9. Top each cupcake with this mixture and refrigerate for 30 minutes before serving.

SMOOTHIE BOWL AS A DESSERT

20 minutes

0 minutes

1 Servings

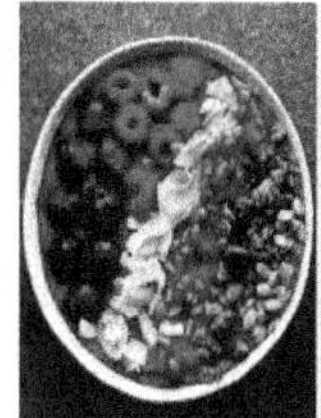
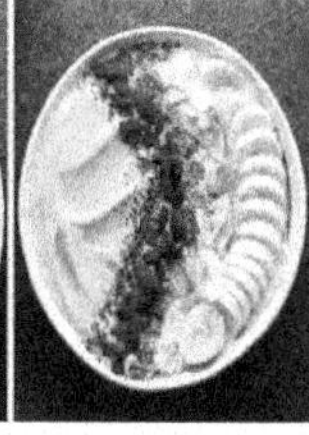

INGREDIENTS

- 100 g frozen strawberries
- 2 bananas
- 2 tbsp pomegranate seeds
- 2 tbsp blueberries
- 1 tbsp sunflower seeds
- 1 tbsp pistachio nuts
- 1 teaspoon bee pollen

COOKING STEPS

1. Let the strawberries thaw 2 hours before preparation.
2. Peel and slice the bananas.
3. Then puree the strawberries with 1 ½ bananas to a homogeneous mass. If this mass is too thick, add a little water.
4. Then divide into bowls.
5. Now decoratively place the remaining banana slices, pomegranate seeds, blueberries, seeds and pollen on top and serve.

AVOCADO AND PASSION FRUIT CREAM WITH PERSIMMON

10 minutes

10 minutes

1 Servings

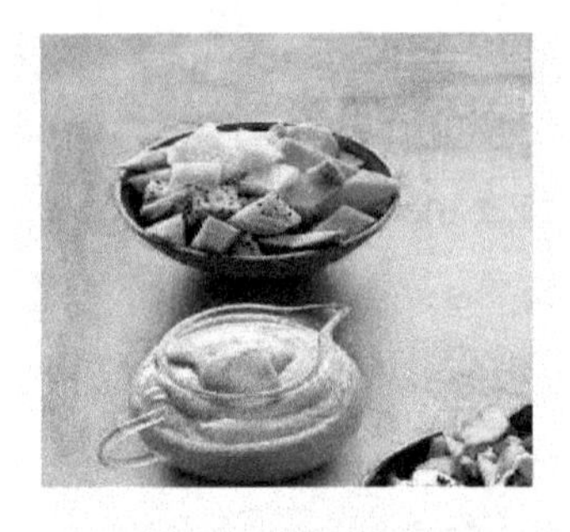

INGREDIENTS

- 1 persimmon
- 1 passion fruit
- ½ avocado
- 2 tbsp almond flakes
- some orange juice

COOKING STEPS

1. Halve and core the avocado and scoop out the pulp.
2. Peel the persimmons and cut and spoon the passion fruit.
3. Put all three ingredients in a blender.
4. Refine with orange juice to taste and then pour the cream into a bowl and serve garnished with the almond flakes.

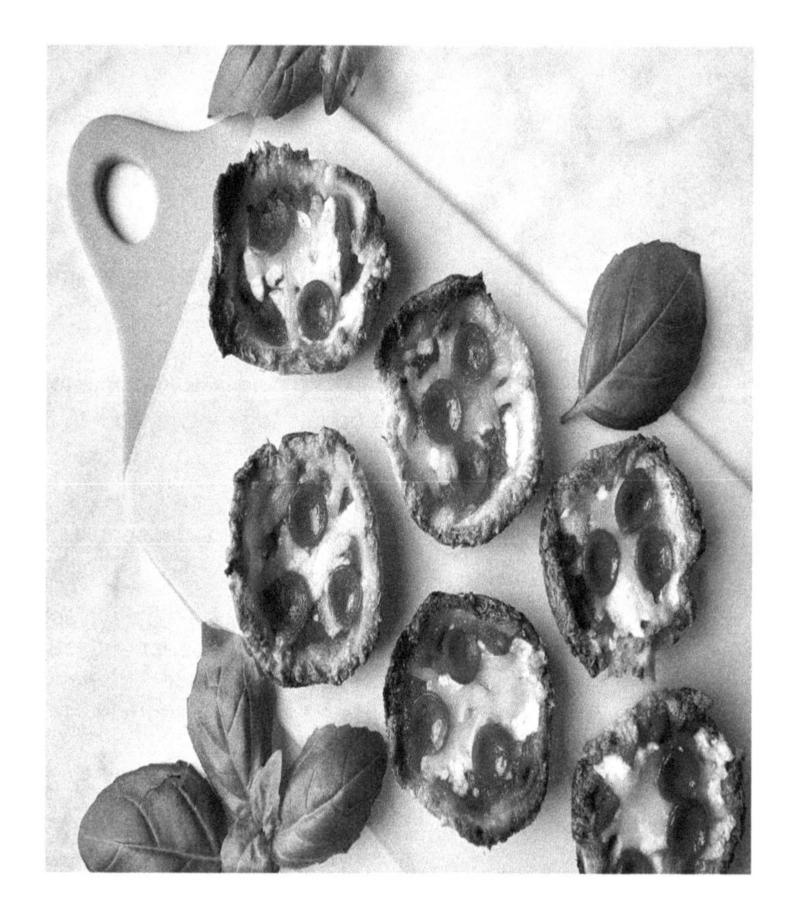

Snack Recipes

BREAD STICKS WITH MUESLI

5 minutes

20 minutes

5 Servings

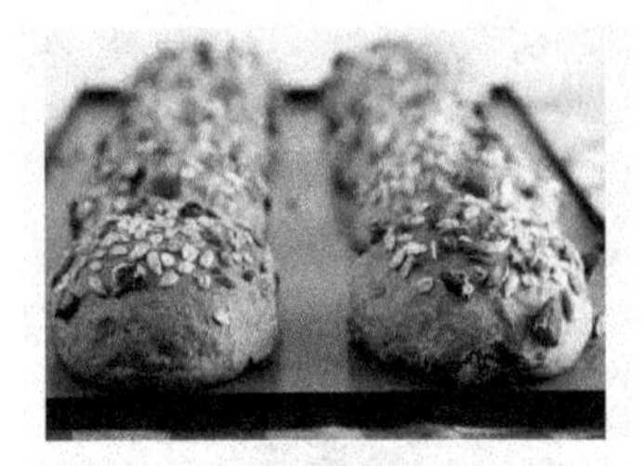

INGREDIENTS

- 200 g of flour
- 10 g fresh yeast
- 250 g low-fat quark
- 1 egg
- 75 g muesli of your choice
- 1 teaspoon salt
- 2 teaspoons of baking powder
- some muesli to sprinkle on

COOKING STEPS

1. Preheat the oven to 200 ° C with top and bottom heat.
2. Mix all ingredients together and use a mixer with kneading dough to mix them together.
3. As soon as smooth dough is formed, the dough can be shaped into 5 sticks.
4. Before these can be put in the oven, they either have to be sprinkled with muesli or rolled in it.
5. Place the sticks on a baking sheet lined with baking paper and let them bake for 15-20 minutes, depending on how dark you want them to be.

MOZZARELLA MOUND SNACKS

5 minutes

10 minutes

3 Servings

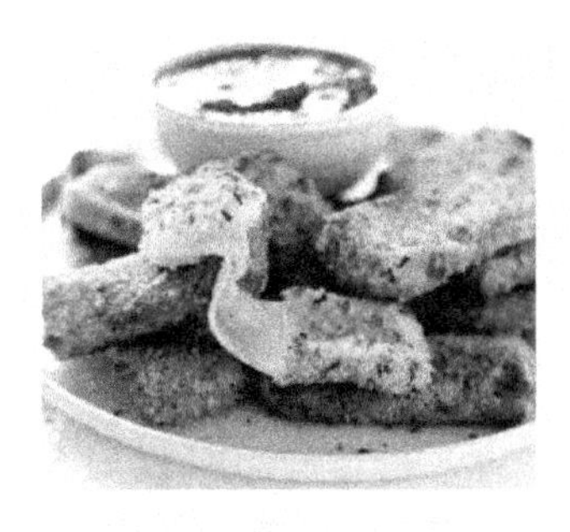

INGREDIENTS

- ⅓ cup of panko bread, flavored with herbs
- 2 egg whites
- 6 tbsp mozzarella cheese, molded into 2 tbsp balls
- ¼ cup marinara sauce

COOKING STEPS

1. Preheat your oven to 425 ° F.
2. Toast the panko breadcrumbs for 2 minutes, stirring frequently, in a medium skillet set over medium heat.
3. Transfer the breadcrumbs to a bowl. Add the egg whites to another bowl.
4. Dip a ball of cheese in the egg and roll it in the panko. Place the breaded cheese on a greased baking sheet and bake for 3 minutes. Repeat the process for the remaining cheese.
5. Heat the marinara sauce in your microwave for half a minute. Serve the breaded cheese ball with the sauce

TASTY TURKEY CHEESE CYLINDERS

5minutes

0 minutes

1 Servings

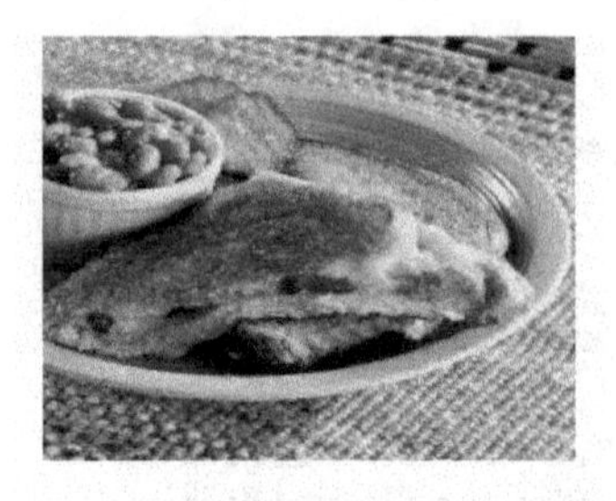

INGREDIENTS

- oz. turkey, roasted and sliced
- 1 oz. cheese

COOKING STEPS

1. Slice the cheese into a long strip, enough to hold the turkey slice.
2. Wrap the slice of turkey around the cheese.

PHILADELPHIA POTATO PRALINE

30 minutes

0 minutes

2 Servings

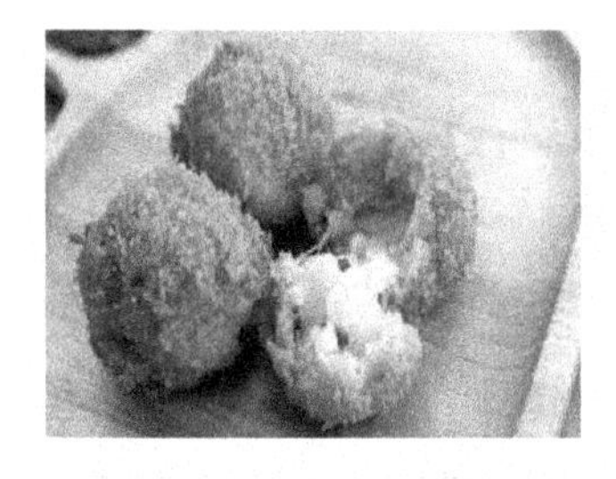

INGREDIENTS

- ⅓ cup Philadelphia Cream Cheese
- 1½ cup unsweetened and grated coconut
- 1 tablespoon of butter
- ¼ teaspoon ground cinnamon
- Sweetener of choice

COOKING STEPS

1. Combine all the ingredients except the ground cinnamon in a bowl.
2. Refrigerate the mixture and let it set until it hardens.
3. Divide the mixture into 8 and roll each serving into potato shapes.
4. Place them on a sheet of baking paper.
5. Sprinkle cinnamon all over and store in the refrigerator for a week before serving.

DREAMY ZUCCHINI BOWL

10 minutes

20 minutes

4 Servings

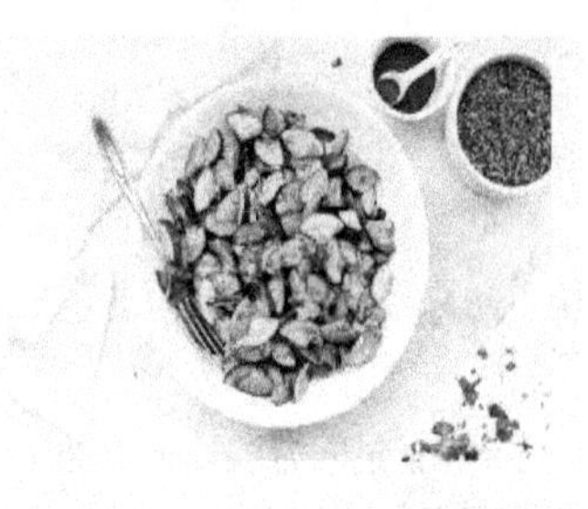

INGREDIENTS

- 1 onion, chopped
- 3 zucchini, cut into medium chunks
- 2 tablespoons coconut almond milk
- 2 garlic cloves, minced
- 4 cups vegetable stock
- 2 tablespoons coconut oil
- Pinch of sunflower seeds
- Black pepper to taste

COOKING STEPS

1. Take a pot and place it over medium heat. Add oil and let it heat up.
2. Add zucchini, garlic, onion, and stir.
3. Cook for 5 minutes.
4. Add stock, sunflower seeds, pepper, and stir. Bring to a boil and reduce heat.
5. Simmer for 20 minutes.
6. Remove from heat and add coconut almond milk. Use an immersion blender until smooth.
7. Ladle into soup bowls and serve. Enjoy!

KIWI AND LIME SMOOTHIE

10 minutes

0 minutes

1 Servings

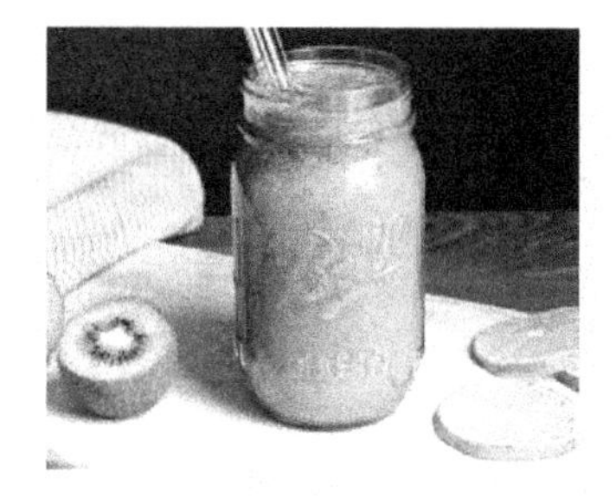

INGREDIENTS

- 1 kiwi
- 1 lime
- 1 tbsp lemon juice
- 1 teaspoon of linseed oil
- 150 ml of still mineral water

COOKING STEPS

1. Please cut and peel the kiwi.
2. Then cut the lime open and put the pulp with the juice in the blender.
3. Add the kiwi and the other ingredients.
4. Then mix everything well.

APPLE CHIPS

10 minutes

5 hours

6 Servings

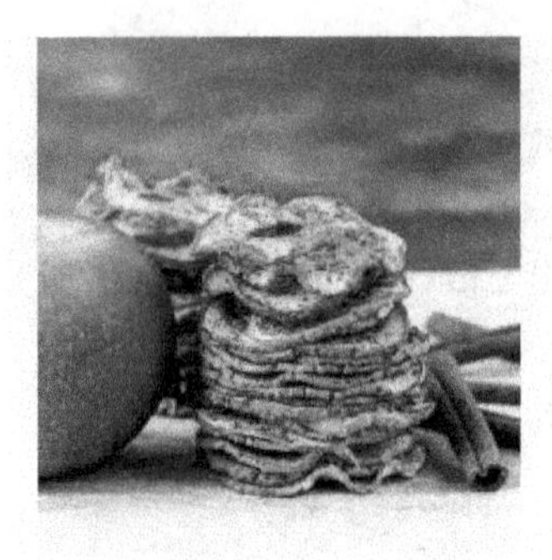

INGREDIENTS

- 2 kg of apples
- 60 ml lemon juice 125 ml of water

COOKING STEPS

1. First, core and peel the apples and cut into thin slices.
2. Mix the water and lemon juice and then turn the apples in it.
3. Preheat the oven to 80 degrees and place the slices in the oven on baking paper.
4. The apples must stay in the oven for 4 hours.

RADICCHIO SALAD

10 minutes

0 minutes

2 Servings

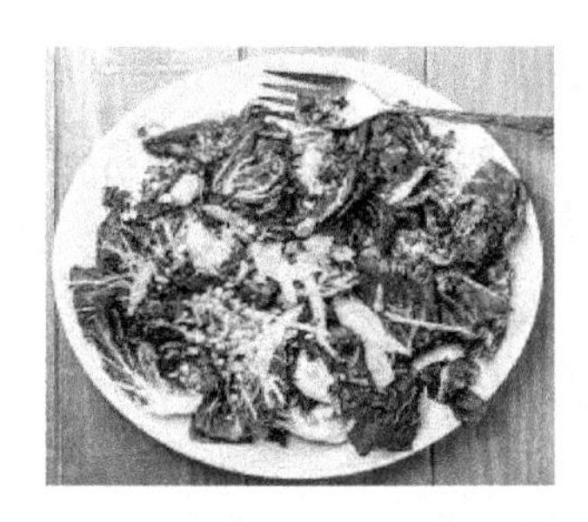

INGREDIENTS

- 1 small radicchio
- 1 bulb of fennel
- 6 halves of a walnut
- 40 g parmesan cheese
- 3 tbsp walnut oil
- 2 tbsp dark balsamic vinegar
- Salt pepper

COOKING STEPS

1. Halve the radicchio and cut out the stalk. Then put the leaves in a large colander and wash them under running water. Then pat dry.
2. Now cut the radicchio into bite-sized pieces and place them in a bowl.
3. Wash the fennel and cut it in half and cut out the stalk in a wedge shape.
4. Now slice the fennel pieces into wafer-thin slices and place them in the bowl.
5. Chop the walnut halves and grate the parmesan.
6. Mix the walnut oil, the balsamic vinegar, and salt and pepper together in a small bowl.
7. Arrange everything accordingly.

CRACKER WITH CHEESE DIP

25 minutes

20 minutes

4 Servings

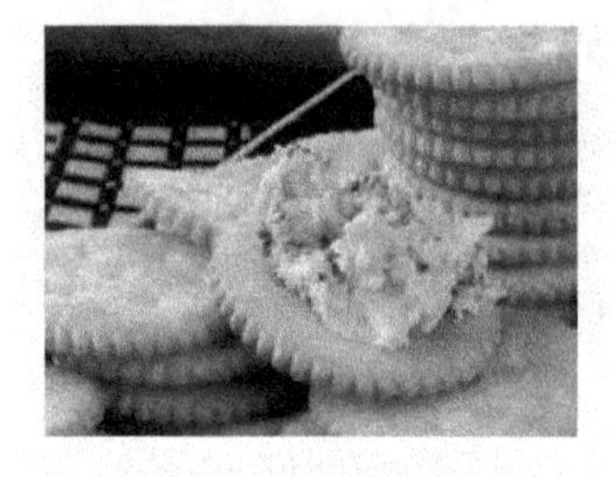

INGREDIENTS

- 150 g cheddar cheese
- 80 g cream cheese
- 75 g of flaxseed
- 75 g pumpkin seeds
- 50 g sesame seeds
- 40g almond flour
- 30 g butter
- 2 tbsp coconut oil
- 2 tbsp milk salt and pepper

COOKING STEPS

1. Put the kernels with the almond flour in a bowl and pour
2. 125 ml of water over them.
3. Then let stand for 10 minutes. Add the coconut oil and season with salt.
4. Then place the mixture on a baking sheet and spread it out. Heat the oven to 175 ° C top and bottom heat and place the tray in the oven for 25 minutes.

ZUCCHINI PAN

5 minutes

10 minutes

1 Servings

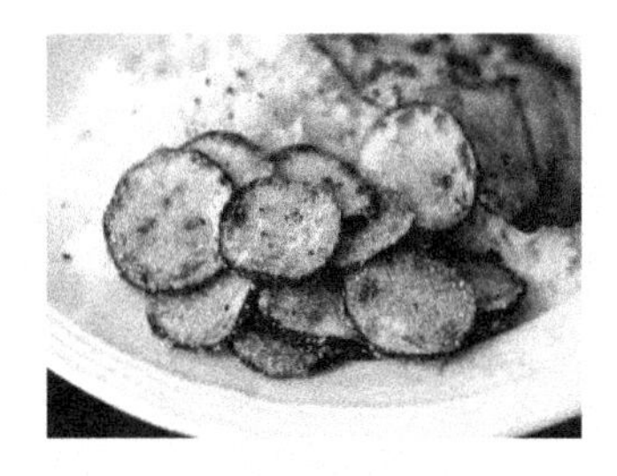

INGREDIENTS

- 1 can of chickpeas
- 220 g drained weight
- 3 medium zucchini
- 1 clove of garlic
- 2 tbsp sesame seeds
- 2 tbsp parsley chopped
- 1 tbsp olive oil
- 1 pinch of cayenne pepper salt and pepper

COOKING STEPS

1. Cut the zucchinis into slices. Heat with oil in a pan and fry for 5 minutes.
2. Meanwhile, pour the chickpeas into a colander and wash them off.
3. Peel and chop the garlic. Then add the chickpeas and garlic to the zucchini slices in the pan.
4. Fry for 5 minutes.
5. At the end add the sesame seeds, herbs and spices, stir and serve.

CPSIA information can be obtained
at www.ICGtesting.com
Printed in the USA
BVHW050801120521
607047BV00003B/395